W9-ARN-395

Every Day Gets
a Little Closer

Every Day Gets a Little Closer

A Twice-Told Therapy

Irvin D. Yalom, M.D.

and

Ginny Elkin

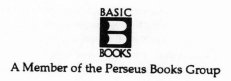

A Member of the Perseus Books Group

Copyright © 1974 by Basic Books, A Member of the Perseus Books Group
Library of Congress Catalog Card Number: 74-78308
ISBN: 465-02119-0 (cloth)
ISBN 0-465-02118-2 (paper)
Manufactured in the United States of America
DESIGNED BY VINCENT TORRE
05 04   RRD   20

Contents

Every Day Gets a Little Closer

Editor's Foreword

IT IS TRUE that the literature of psychotherapy already numbers many works which recount the saga of recovery. Since the turn of the century, psychiatrists have increasingly elected to publish illustrative and exceptional case histories, and, not to be outdone, patients have increasingly presented their own retrospective versions. This book is unique in that it simultaneously traces the course of treatment from the vantage points of both patient and doctor, as they evolve a delicate and difficult relationship which has personal meaning for both of them.

The book is an outgrowth of an experiment undertaken by my husband, Dr. Irvin Yalom of Stanford University, and one of his patients, henceforth known as Ginny. In the fall of 1970 my husband decided that it would be inadvisable for Ginny to continue with him and a co-therapist in group therapy, since she had made virtually no progress in that format for a year and a half, and he suggested that they subsequently meet in individual therapy. Because Ginny's problems included that of a "writer's block" (a serious complaint for an aspiring novelist), Dr. Yalom stipulated that she pay for treatment in the form of post-session reports, which would provide an obvious stimulus to her writing. At the same time Dr. Yalom decided that he too would prepare a separate account of their weekly meetings, with the understanding that he and Ginny would exchange these reports at six months' intervals, in the hope of therapeutic benefit. For two years thereafter doctor and patient recorded his and her recollections of the hour they had shared together, frequently adding afterthoughts, interpretations, emotions and associations which hadn't been voiced during the session.

Although my husband almost never discusses his patients with me, I was privy to some of his reflections on Ginny as he considered this method of encouraging her writing. Since I am a professor of literature, he knew this project would be of real interest to me. I suggested that he carefully preserve both sets of reports until the end of therapy and then decide whether they merited a wider audience.

Privately I wondered if the post-session reports might not constitute a publishable piece of literature, with two distinct characters and two recognizable literary styles, not unlike an epistolary novel.

It was, thus, with an especial interest that I read the manuscript for the first time two years later. My enthusiastic evaluation, and that of less biased judges, succeeded in persuading the authors to publish it. Although changes were necessary to conceal the identity of the patient and to adapt the doctor's tapescripts for a reading public, the words are essentially those of the original texts. No supplemental thoughts or fictive events have been added to the symbiotic drama of psychotherapy. In the case of the doctor's accounts, not one significant reflection has been added or omitted—except for a few tapes which were, unfortunately, mislaid and lost for good. Aside from very minor stylistic corrections, Ginny's reports are virtually unaltered.

At the suggestion of several readers who found the manuscript difficult to approach without some explanatory material, and others who were eager to know what became of Ginny after therapy, Dr. Yalom and Ginny each wrote a Foreword and an Afterword composed a year and a half after their last therapeutic meeting together. These do add considerable information and clarification of both a personal and theoretical nature. Still, it is my belief that the central portion can be read like a novel, as the story of two human beings who met in the intimacy of the psychiatric tête-à-tête and now permit you to know them as they knew each other.

Marilyn Yalom
February 20, 1974

Doctor Yalom's Foreword

IT ALWAYS wrenches me to find old appointment books filled with the half forgotten names of patients with whom I have had the most tender experiences. So many people, so many fine moments. What has happened to them? My many-tiered file cabinets, my mounds of tape recordings often remind me of some vast cemetery: lives pressed into clinical folders, voices trapped on electromagnetic bands mutely and eternally playing out their dramas. Living with these monuments imbues me with a keen sense of transience. Even as I find myself immersed in the present I sense the specter of decay watching and waiting—a decay which will ultimately vanquish lived experience and yet, by its very inexorability, bestows a poignancy and beauty. The desire to relate my experience with Ginny is a very compelling one; I am intrigued by the opportunity to stave off decay, to prolong the span of our brief life together. How much better to know that it will exist in the mind of the reader rather than in the abandoned warehouse of unread clinical notes and unheard electromagnetic tapes.

The story begins with a phone call. A thready voice told me that her name was Ginny, that she had just arrived in California, that she had been in therapy for several months with a colleague of mine in the East who had referred her to me. Having recently returned from a year's sabbatical in London, I had still much free time and scheduled a meeting with Ginny two days later.

I met her in the waiting room and ushered her down the hall into my office. I could not walk slowly enough; like an Oriental wife she followed a few noiseless steps behind. She did not belong to herself, nothing went with anything else—her hair, her grin, her voice, her walk, her sweater, her shoes, everything had been flung together by chance, and there was the immediate possibility of all—hair, walk, limbs, tattered jeans, G.I. socks, everything—flying asunder. Leaving what? I wondered. Perhaps just the grin. Not pretty, no matter how one arranged the parts! Yet curiously appealing. Somehow, in only minutes, she managed to let me know that I could do everything and that she completely delivered herself up into my hands. I did not mind. At the time it did not seem a heavy burden.

She spoke, and I learned that she was twenty-three years old, the daughter of a one-time opera singer and a Philadelphia businessman. She had a sister four years younger and a gift for creative writing. She had come to California because she had been accepted, on the basis of some short stories, into a one-year creative writing program at a nearby college.

Why was she now seeking help? She said that she needed to continue the therapy she had begun last year, and, in a confusing unsystematic fashion, gradually recounted her major difficulties in living. In addition to her explicit complaints, I recognized during the course of the interview several other major problem areas.

First, her self-portrait—related quickly and breathlessly with occasional fetching metaphors punctuating the litany of self-hatred. She is masochistic in all things. All her life she has neglected her own needs and pleasures. She has no respect for herself. She feels she is a disembodied spirit—a chirping canary hopping back and forth from shoulder to shoulder, as she and her friends walk down the street. She imagines that only as an ethereal wisp is she of interest to others.

She has no sense of herself. She says, "I have to prepare myself to be with people. I plan what I am going to say. I have no spontaneous feelings—I do, but within some little cage. Whenever I go outside I feel fearful and must prepare myself." She does not recognize or express her anger. "I am full of pity for people. I am that walking cliché: 'If you can't say anything nice about people, don't say anything at all.'" She remembers getting angry only once in her adult life: years ago she yelled at a coworker who was insolently ordering her around. She trembled for hours afterward. She has no rights. It doesn't occur to her to be angry. She is so totally absorbed with making others like her that she never thinks of asking herself whether she likes others.

She is consumed with self-contempt. A small voice inside endlessly taunts her. Should she forget herself for a moment and engage life spontaneously, the pleasure-stripping voice brings her back sharply to her casket of self-consciousness. In the interview she could not permit herself a single prideful sentiment. No sooner had she mentioned her creative writing program than she rushed to remind me that she had come by it through sloth; hearing about this program through gossip, she had applied for it only because it required no formal application other than sending in some stories she had written two years previously. Of course, she did not comment on the presumably high quality of the stories. Her literary output had gradually waned and she was now in the midst of a severe writing block.

All of her problems in living were reflected in her relationships with men. Though she desperately wanted a lasting relationship with a man, she had never been able to sustain one. At the age of twenty-one she leapt from nubile sexual innocence to sexual intercourse with several men (she had no right to say "no!") and lamented that she had hurled herself through the bedroom window without even entering the adolescent antechamber of dating and petting. She enjoys being physically close to a man but cannot release herself sexually. She has experienced orgasm through masturbation, but the internal taunting voice makes quite certain that she rarely approaches orgasm in sexual intercourse.

Ginny rarely mentioned her father but her mother's presence was very large. "I am my mother's pale reflection," she put it. They have always been unusually close. Ginny told her mother everything. She remembers how she and mother used to read and chuckle over Ginny's love letters. Ginny was always thin, had many food aversions and for over a year in her early teens vomited so regularly before breakfast that her family grew to consider it as part of her routine morning toilet. She always ate a great deal, but when she was very young she could swallow only with much difficulty. "I would eat a whole meal and at the end still have it all in my mouth. I would try then to swallow it all at once."

She has horrible nightmares in which she is sexually violated, usually by a woman, but sometimes by a man. Also a recurrent dream in which either she is a large breast with clusters of people clinging to her or she herself clings to some mammoth breast. About three years ago she began having frightening dreams where it was difficult for her to ascertain if she were asleep or awake. She senses people staring at her through the window and touching her; as soon as she starts to experience pleasure from the touching, it turns to pain as though her breasts are being tugged off. Throughout all of these dreams there is a far away voice reminding her that none of this is really happening.

By the end of the hour I felt considerable alarm about Ginny. Despite many strengths—a soft charm, deep sensitivity, wit, a highly developed comic sense, a remarkable gift for verbal imagery—I found pathology wherever I turned: too much primitive material, dreams which obscured the reality-fantasy border, but above all a strange diffuseness, a blurring of "ego boundaries." She seemed incompletely differentiated from her mother, and her feeding problems suggested a feeble and pathetic attempt at liberation. I experienced her as feeling trapped between the terrors of an infantile dependency which required a relinquishment of selfhood—a permanent stagnation—and, on the other hand, an assumption of an autonomy which, without a deep sense of self, seemed stark and unbearably lonely.

I rarely trouble myself excessively with diagnosis. But I know that because of her ego boundary blurring, her autism, her dream life, the inaccessibility of affect, most clinicians would affix to her a label of "schizoid" or, perhaps, "borderline." I knew that she was seriously troubled and that therapy would be long and chancy. It seemed to me that she had too much familiarity already with her unconscious and that I must guide her to reality rather than escort her more deeply into her underworld. I was at that moment hurriedly forming a therapy group which my students were to observe as part of their training program, and since my experience in group therapy with individuals who have problems similar to Ginny's has been good, I decided to offer her a place in the group. She accepted the recommendation a bit reluctantly; she liked the idea of being with others but feared that she would become a child in the group and never be able to express her intimate thoughts. This is a typical expectation of a new patient in group therapy, and I reassured her that, as her trust in the group developed, she would be able to share her feelings with the others. Unfortunately, as we shall see, her prediction of her behavior proved all too accurate.

Aside from the practical consideration of my forming a group and searching for patients, I had reservations about treating Ginny individually. In particular I felt some disquiet at the depth of her admiration for me, which, like some ready-made mantle, was thrust over me as soon as she entered my office. Consider her dream dreamt the night before our first meeting. "I had severe diarrhea and a man was going to buy me some medicine that had Rx's written on it. I kept thinking I should have Kaopectate because it was cheaper, but he wanted to buy me the most expensive medicine possible." Some of the positive feelings for me stemmed from her previous therapist's high praise of me, some from my professorial title, the rest from parts unknown. But the overevaluation was so extreme that I suspected it would prove an impediment in individual therapy. Participation in group therapy, I reasoned, would allow Ginny the opportunity to view me through the eyes of many individuals. Furthermore, the presence of a co-therapist in the group should allow her to obtain a more balanced view of me.

During the first month of the group Ginny did very poorly. Terrifying nightmares interrupted her sleep nightly. For example, she dreamt that her teeth were glass and her mouth had turned to blood. Another dream reflected some of her feelings about sharing me with the group. "I was lying prostrate on the beach, and was picked up and carried away to a doctor who was to perform an operation on my brain. The doctor's hands were held and so guided by two of the group members that he accidently cut a part of the brain he hadn't intended to." Another dream involved her going to a party with me and our rolling on the grass together in sexual play.

After the first month my co-therapist and I both felt that a once-a-week group was not enough for Ginny and that some supportive individual therapy was necessary, both to prevent Ginny from decompensating even further and to help her pass through the difficult early stage of the group. She expressed a wish to see me individually, but I felt that it would be more complicating than helpful to see her both individually and in a group and thus referred her to another psychiatrist in our clinic. She saw him individually twice a week for approximately nine months and continued to attend the group therapy meetings for approximately eighteen months. Her individual therapist noted that Ginny was "beleaguered by frightening masochistic sexual fantasies and manifestly borderline schizophrenic thought processes." He attempted in his therapy to be "ego-supportive and to focus on reality testing and distortions in her interpersonal relationships."

Ginny attended the group religiously, rarely missing a meeting even when after one year she moved to San Francisco which necessitated a long inconvenient commute via public transportation. Though Ginny received enough support from the group to hold her own during this time, she made no real progress. In fact, few patients would have shown the perseverance to continue so long in the group with so little benefit. There was reason to believe that Ginny continued in the group primarily to continue her contact with me. She persisted in her conviction that I, and perhaps only I, had the power to help her. Repeatedly the therapists and the group members made this observation; repeatedly they noted that Ginny was fearful of changing since improvement would mean that she would lose me. Only by remaining fixed in her helpless state could she insure my presence. But there was no movement. She remained tense, withdrawn and often noncommunicative in the group. The other members were intrigued by her; when she did speak, she was often perceptive and helpful to others. One of the men in the group fell deeply in love with her, and others vied for her attention. But the thaw never came, she remained frozen with terror and never was able to express her feelings freely or to interact with the others.

During the eighteen months Ginny was in the group I had two co-therapists, each male, each remaining with the group for approximately nine months. Their observations about Ginny closely parallel my own: "ethereal . . . wistful . . . a haughty but self-conscious amusement at the whole proceedings . . . reality would never fully engage her energies. . . . A 'presence' in the group . . . a tortured transference to Dr. Yalom which withstood all interpretative efforts . . . everything she did in the group was considered in the light of his approval or disapproval . . . alternated between being someone who was extraordinarily sensitive and reactive to others, to someone who simply was not there at all . . . a mystery in the group . . . a borderline schizophrenic yet she never came close to the border of psychosis . . . schizoid . . . too much awareness of primary process . . ."

During the period of her group therapy, Ginny searched for other methods to escape from the dungeon of self-consciousness she had constructed for herself. She frequently attended Esalen and other local growth centers. The leaders of these programs designed a number of crash-program confrontational techniques to change Ginny instantaneously: nude marathons to overcome her reserve and hiddenness, psychodrama techniques and psychological karate to alter her meekness and unassertiveness, and vaginal stimulation with an electric vibrator to awake her slumbering orgasm. All to no avail! She was an excellent actress and could easily assume another role on stage. Unfortunately, when the performance was over she shed her new role quickly and left the theater clad as she had entered it.

Ginny's fellowship at college ended, her savings dwindled and she had to find work. Finally, a part-time job provided an irreconcilable scheduling conflict, and Ginny, after agonized weeks of deliberation, served notice that she would have to leave the group. At approximately the same time my co-therapist and I had concluded that there was little likelihood of her benefiting from the group. I met with her to discuss future plans. It was apparent that she required continued therapy; though her grasp on reality was more firm, the monstrous night and waking dreams had abated, she was living with a young man, Karl (of whom we shall hear more later), and had formed a small group of friends, she enjoyed life still with only a small fraction of her energies. Her internal demon, a pleasure-stripping small voice, tormented her relentlessly and she continued to live her life against a horizon of dread and self-consciousness. The relationship to Karl, the closest she had ever experienced, was a particular source of agony. Though she cared deeply for him, she was convinced that his feelings toward her were so conditional that any foolish word or false move would tip the balance against her. Consequently, she derived little pleasure from the creature comforts she shared with Karl.

I considered referring Ginny for individual therapy to a public clinic in San Francisco (she could not afford to see a therapist in private practice), but many doubts nagged me. The waiting lists were long, the therapists sometimes inexperienced. But the compelling factor was that Ginny's great faith in me colluded with my rescuer fantasy to convince me that only I could save her. Besides all this I have a very stubborn streak; I hate to give up and admit that I cannot help a patient.

So I did not surprise myself when I offered to continue treating Ginny. I wanted, however, to break the set. A number of therapists had failed to help her and I looked for an approach which would not repeat the errors of the others and at the same time permit me to capitalize, for therapeutic benefit, on Ginny's powerful positive transference to me. I describe in some detail my therapeutic plan and the theoretical rationale underlying my approach in the Afterword. For now, I need only comment on one aspect of the approach, a bold procedural ploy which has resulted in the following pages. I asked Ginny, in lieu of financial payment, to write an honest summary of each session, containing not only her reactions to what transpired, but also a depiction of the subterranean life of the hour, a note from the underground—all the thoughts and fantasies that never emerged into the daylight of verbal intercourse. I thought the idea, innovative to the best of my knowledge in psychotherapeutic practice, was a happy one; Ginny was then so inert that any technique demanding effort and motion seemed worth trying. Ginny's total writing block which deprived her of an important source of positive self-regard made a procedure requiring mandatory writing even more appealing. (Incidentally, this plan entailed no personal financial sacrifice since I was on a full-time salary status with Stanford University and any money I earned from clinical work was turned over to the University.)

Because of my wife's interest in literature and the creative process, I mentioned this plan to her and she suggested that I, too, write an impressionistic nonclinical note following each session. I thought this idea was an inspired one, though for an entirely different reason from that of my wife: she was interested in the literary aspect of the endeavor; I, on the other hand, was intrigued by a potentially powerful exercise in self-disclosure. Ginny could not disclose herself to me, or anyone, in a face-to-face encounter. She regarded me as infallible, omniscient, untroubled, perfectly integrated. I imagined her sending me, in a letter if you will, her unspoken wishes and feelings toward me. I imagined her reading my own personal and deeply fallible messages to her. I could not know the precise effects of the exercise, but I felt certain that the plan would release something powerful.

I knew that our writing would be inhibited if we were conscious of the other's immediate perusal; so we agreed not to read the other's reports for several months and my secretary would store them for us. Artificial? Contrived? We would see. I knew that the arena of therapy and of change would be the relationship existing between us. I believed that if we could, one day, replace the letters with words immediately spoken to one another, that if we could relate in an honest, human fashion, then all other desired changes would follow.

Ginny's Foreword

I WAS an A student in high school in New York. Even though I was creative, that was just a sideline to being mostly stunned, as though I had been hit on the head by a monster shyness. I went through puberty with my eyes shut and my head migrained. Fairly early in my college life I put myself out to pasture academically. Although I did occasional "great" work, I liked nothing better than to be a human sundial, a curled up outdoor nap. I was scared of boys and didn't have any. My few later affairs were all surprises. As part of my college education, I spent some time in Europe working and studying and compiling a dramatic résumé that was really all anecdotes and friends, not progress. What passed for bravery was a form of nervous energy and inertia. I was scared to come home.

After I graduated from college, I returned to New York. I couldn't find a job, in fact had no direction. My qualifications dripped like Dali's watch, as I was tempted toward everything and nothing. By chance, I got a job teaching small children. Actually none of the children (and there were only about eight) were pupils; they were kindred spirits and what we did was play for a year.

While in New York I took classes in acting on how to howl and breathe and read lines so they sounded like they were hooked up to a real blood stream. There was a stillness to my life though, no matter how much I rushed through classes and friends.

Even when I didn't know what I was doing, I smiled a great deal. One friend, feeling himself pressed up against Pollyanna, said, "What have you got to be so happy about?" In fact, with my few great friends (I've always had them), I could be happy; my faults seemed only minor distractions compared to how natural and easy life was. However, my grin was stifling. My mind was filled with a jangling carousel of words that rotated constantly around moods and aromas, only occasionally dropping out into my voice or onto paper. I was not too good when it came to facts. I lived alone in New York. My contact with the outside world, except for classes and letters, was minimal. I began to masturbate for the first time, and found it frightening, just because it was something private happening in my life. The transparent quality of my fears and happiness had always made me feel light and silly. A friend said, "I can read you like a book." I was someone like Puck, who didn't need any responsibility; who never did anything more serious than vomit. And suddenly I was starting to act differently. Quickly I began to immerse myself in therapy.

The therapist was a woman and in the five months I was with her, twice a week, she tried to make my grin go away. She was convinced that my whole objective in therapy was to get her to like me. In the sessions she pounded away at my relationship with my parents. It had always been ridiculously loving and open and ironic.

I was afraid in therapy because I was sure there was some horrible secret that my mind was withholding from me. Some explanation of why my life felt like one of those children's drawing boards: when you lift up the paper, the easy funny faces, the squiggly lines, are all erased, leaving no traces. At that time no matter how much I did, how many best friends I loved, I was dependent on others to give me my setting and pulse. I was both vibrant and dead. I needed their push; I could never be self-starting. And my memory was mostly deadly and derogatory.

I was progressing in therapy to the point where both me and my feelings were sitting in the same leather chair. Then an unusual circumstance changed my life, or at least my location. I had applied on a whim to a writing program in California and was accepted. My therapist in New York was not happy with the news; in fact, was against my going. She said I was stuck, took no responsibility for my life, and no amount of fellowship was going to get me out. However, I could not act adult about it and write to the grant people saying, "Please postpone my miraculous stipend while I try to find my emotions and feel confident and human." No, like everything else, I waded into the new environment, even though I was afraid that my therapist's words were correct and that I was just leaving at the beginning, risking my life for a guaranteed year of sun. But I could not refuse experience, since that was my alibi, my backdrop for feeling, my way of thinking, of moving. Always the scenic view rather than the serious, thoughtful route.

My therapist in the end gave me her blessing, convinced that I could get excellent help from a psychiatrist she knew in California. I left New York, and as always there was something thrilling about leaving. No matter how many valuables you have left behind, you still have your energy and your eyes, and right before I left, my grin, like a permanent logo, came back, with the exhilaration of getting out. I gambled that the psychological pot would still be waiting for me when I arrived in California, and I wouldn't have to start from scratch as a child star.

Because of the intensive and heroic work I had done in New York with acting, therapy and loneliness, I made it to California with all my limited, padded feelings still intact. It was a great time in my life because I had a guaranteed future, plus no men whom I had to try and stretch myself for and be judged by. I hadn't had any boyfriend since college. I found a small cottage with an orange tree in front; I never even thought of picking the oranges off the tree till a friend said I could. I substituted tennis for acting. And made my usual quota of one great girlfriend. At the college I did okay, though I acted like an ingenue.

I went from one therapist to another in coming from New York to Mountain View.

In a teetering frame of mind, teething on Chekhov and Jacques Brel and other sweet and sour sadnesses, I first went to see Dr. Yalom. Expectations, which are an important part of my lot, were great since he had been recommended by my New York therapist. As I went into his room vulnerable and warm, maybe even Bela Lugosi could have done the trick, but I doubt it. Dr. Yalom was special.

That first interview with him, my soul became infatuated. I could talk straight; I could cry, I could ask for help and not be ashamed. There were no recriminations waiting to escort me home. All his questions seemed to penetrate past the mush of my brain. Coming into his room I seemed to have license to be myself. I trusted Dr. Yalom. He was Jewish—and that day, I was too. He seemed familiar and natural without being a Santa Claus psychiatrist type.

Dr. Yalom suggested I join his group therapy that he conducted with another doctor. It was like signing up for the wrong course—I wanted Poetry and Religion on a one-to-one visitation and instead I got beginning bridge (and with no good chocolate mix either). He sent me to the co-leader of the group. In my preliminary interview with the other doctor there were no tears, no truths, just the subtext of an impersonal tape recorder breathing.

Group therapy is really hard. Especially if the table is stacked with inertia as ours was. The group of about seven patients plus two doctors met at a round table with a microphone dangling from the ceiling; on one side there was a wall of mirrors like a glassy web where my face would get caught every once in awhile looking at itself. A group of resident doctors sat on the other side and looked in the window mirror. It really didn't bother me. Although I am shy, I am also a little exhibitionist, and I removed myself accordingly and "acted" like a stuffed Ophelia. The table and chair put you in a posture where it was difficult to get going.

Many of us had the same problems—an inability to feel, unjelled anger, love troubles. There were a few miraculous days when one or the other of us caught fire and something would happen. But the time boundaries on either side of the hour and a half usually doused any big breakthroughs. And by the next week we had subsided into our usual psychological rigor mortis. (I should speak for myself. Others did get helped a lot.) In the group it was fun to share problems but we rarely shared solutions. We became friends; we never touched (which is practically a given in California). Toward the end we went out for pizzas with everything on them. I enjoyed Dr. Yalom as a group leader even as I became more distant and lop-sided, hardly ever interacting with him, except visually. Part of my problem was that as usual I wasn't making decisions in my personal life, but drifting by on presence and friends. I couldn't really hold my head up. (I had a few months of private therapy concurrent with group therapy. It was with a young doctor. I'd been having horrible dreams and Dr. Yalom had suggested it.)

I was beginning to feel lifeless again and pretentious, so I sought artificial respiration from encounter groups, which were indigenous to the area. They were held in people's lush forest homes—on rugs, on straw mats, in Japanese baths, at midnight. I enjoyed the milieu even more than the content. Physicists, dancers, middle-aged people, boxers would show up with their skills and problems. There would be stage lights and Bob Dylan coaching from the corner of a hi-fi, you *know* something is happening, but you don't know what it is.

This form of theater with your soul auditioning appealed to me. There were tears and screaming and laughter and silence—all energizing. Fear, real hits on the back and friendships staggered up out of the midnight slime. Marriages dissolved before your eyes; white collar jobs were slashed. I gladly signed up for these judgment days and resurrections since I'd had nothing like it in my life.

Sometimes you would only be brought down though, without any upward sweep and salvation. You were supposed to be able to follow a certain ritual rhythm and beat, from fear and panic to howling insight, confession and acclamation. And if that failed you were supposed to be able to say, "Well, I'm a schmuck, I'm hopeless, so what? I'm going to go on from there," and dance out your stomach cramps.

Eventually though I realized I was straddling two opposite salvations—the impacted, solid, sluggish, constant, patient group therapy which was just like my life; and the medieval carnivals of the mind and heart of the psychodramas. I knew Dr. Yalom disapproved of my encounters, especially one particular group leader who was inspired and brilliant but with no credentials other than magic. I never really chose my side but continued both forms of therapy, diminishing all the while. Finally in group therapy I got to feel as though I dragged my cocoon in, fastened it onto the chair each week, held on for an hour and a half and left. Refusing to be born.

I was bloated from the many months of group therapy, but was making no move to get out of the situation. My life was happy and yet as usual I felt somewhat submerged and foggy. Through friends I'd met a boyfriend named Karl who was intelligent and dynamic. He had his own book business, which I helped him with, learning no skills but managing to ply him with my jokes and getting stirred up inside. I was at first, however, not naturally attracted to him, which worried me. There was something about his eyes that seemed a little fierce and alien. But I enjoyed being with him even though I had some doubts, because unlike my few other loves, Karl was not an immediate crush, not someone I would have chosen from afar.

After a few terrific weeks of dalliance, we settled into a livable nonchalance. One day, almost as an aside, he told me there was an apartment he knew of where we could live together, and I moved from Mountain View into the city. Karl once said, holding me, that I brought humanity into his life, but he wasn't given to many love declarations.

We began living together easily and enjoying ourselves. It was the beginning of our life together and there were plenty of new green shoots—movies, books, walks, talks, embraces, meals, making our friends mutual and giving up some. I remember I had a physical around then at a free clinic and they wrote: "A twenty-five-year-old, white female in excellent health."

I had left psychodrama by then, and the group therapy was just a habit that I dared not give up. I was waiting as usual to see what would happen in therapy rather than choose my own fate. One day Dr. Yalom called and asked if I would like to have private, free therapy with him on condition that we would both write about it afterward. It was one of those wonderful calls from out of the blue that I am susceptible to. I said yes, overjoyed.

When I began therapy as a private patient with Dr. Yalom, two years had gone by since my first fertile interview with him. I had replaced acting with tennis, looking for someone with being with someone, experiencing loneliness to trying to recall it. Inside I had a feeling that I had skipped out on my problems and that they would all be waiting for me at the ambush of night, some night. The critics, such as my New York therapist, and loves, whom I carried around with me would have said that there was hard work to be done. That I had succeeded too easily without deserving it, and that Karl, who had started calling me "babe," really didn't know my name. I tried to get him to call me by my name—Ginny—and whenever he did my life flowed. Sometimes, though, in deference to my blond hair and nerves, he called me the Golden Worrier.

Eighteen months of hibernation in group therapy had left me groggy and soiled. I began private therapy with only vague anxieties.

I

The First Fall

(October 9–December 9)

DR. YALOM

GINNY appeared today in, what is for her, relatively good shape. Her clothes have no patches on them, her hair has possibly been brushed, her face seems less broken out and far more in focus. With some awkwardness, she described how my suggestion to pay for sessions with write-ups rather than money had given her a new lease on life. At first she had felt elated, but then managed to undercut her optimism by making sarcastic jokes about herself to other people. When asked what kind of sarcastic jokes they were, she said I would probably publish our write-ups under the title of "interviews with an ambulatory catatonic patient." Wanting to clarify our arrangement, I assured her that whatever we wrote would be joint property and if we published anything, we would do it together. I told her it was premature and something that I hadn't really considered (a lie, since I have had flitting fantasies of publishing this material some day).

Then I tried to focus things a bit, lest we wander endlessly in the haze so characteristic of time with Ginny. What did she want to work on in therapy with me? Where did she hope to "go"? She responded by describing her life now as generally empty and meaningless; the most pressing problem is her difficulty with sex. I urged her to be more explicit and she described how she could never allow herself to let go just when she sensed she was at the point of orgasm. The more she talked, the more she struck up chords within me of some conversations I have recently had with Viktor Frankl (a prominent existential analyst). She spends so much time thinking about sex when she is in the midst of it, asking herself what she can do to bring herself off, that she inhibits any possible spontaneity. I thought of ways I might help de-reflect her and finally came out quite artlessly with, "if only there were some way you could de-reflect yourself." She reminded me of the centipede in a children's book who, when asked to watch the way he walks, can no longer manage his hundred pairs of legs.

When I asked her what her day was like, Ginny talked about how empty time was for her, beginning with the emptiness of writing in the morning, which led into the emptiness of the rest of the day. I wondered with her why the writing was so empty and what there was that gave her meaning in life. More shades of Viktor Frankl! So often now recent readings or conversations with other therapists creep into my therapy, which makes me feel like a chameleon with no color of my own.

Later it happened again. I commented to her that her whole life was played out against soft background music of self-abnegation. There was an echo of what a Kleinian * analyst once told me years ago when I considered entering analysis with him: that the analysis would be carried out against the background music of my skepticism of his theoretic position.

In a thread-like voice Ginny continued to present herself as a person lacking both propulsion and direction. She is drawn to emptiness like a magnet and sucks it up and spits it out in front of me. One would think that nothing in her life exists except nothingness. For example, she described sending some stories to *Mademoiselle* and receiving an encouraging letter from the editor. When I asked her when she had gotten the letter, she told me that it was only a few days ago; I remarked that it could have happened years ago from the apathetic tone of her voice. It's the same when she speaks about Eve, a very good friend, or Karl, her boyfriend with whom she lives. There is this little demon within Ginny stealing the meaning and pleasure from everything she does. At the same time she tends to observe herself and romanticize her plight in a tragic way. She flirts, I think, with the vision of herself as a Virginia Woolf who one day will fill her pockets with rocks and walk into the ocean.

Her expectations from me are so unrealistic, she sees me in such an idealized way that I feel discouraged, sometimes hopeless, of ever really making contact with her. I wonder if I'm not exploiting her by asking her to write these reports. Maybe I am. I rationalize it by saying that at least it forces her to write, and I do feel strongly that after six months, when we exchange these notes, something good will come of it. If nothing else, Ginny will have to begin to see me in a different way.

---

* A London-based analytic school founded upon the teachings of Melanie Klein.

October 9

GINNY

THERE must be a way to tell about the session other than repeating exactly what happened and mesmerizing myself and you. I had built up expectations, but I concentrated mostly on thinking of the change in time schedule. I started and ended the session with that busy thought. Fussing and not feeling.

I felt like a dilettante in your office, at first. You were asking me what was on the agenda, what I wanted to happen. I have a long history of not answering or taking questions seriously. I never use my mind or cast it out further than the present, except when I use it to fantasize. I don't let it change or shape reality, just comment on its passing. Your insistence, though, when you kept repeating the question, "Well, what does it mean—your writing not going any-where?" finally annoyed me. It was like a countdown in a fight. I knew I had to get up at that point, and say something or it was all over. After three or four repeats of that question, I said: "What I guess I feel is that it's not the writing, it's the judgment thing in me that doesn't go anywhere, that stays pointing to zero, fluctuating slightly in either direction when there is applause or criticism." I never let on, when I was talking about Karl and me in such a grey voice, that Sunday and Monday mornings had been lovely, with great tenderness and playfulness. Why did I misrepresent myself? (My father's favorite criticism: "All your life you've downgraded yourself, Ginny.") But why couldn't I come in and tell you some good things, especially since I know you like to hear them?

When I was talking to you I was conscious of trying to remember what I had said the time before. I wanted to be sure I didn't repeat myself in this session. At the end, though, I thought I had.

I didn't want to go in and talk about sex since that always sounds so Ann Landers and mature and impersonal. And besides, the im-portance of sex happens with me not in the sometimes good, some-times bad, act but the reprisal the moment after. The occasion to hate myself and fear punishment and recognition from someone else and try to cope with the full-length darkness and conscience.

5

When you used the word "de-reflect" so calmly I liked that a lot. (Afterwards I used the word in three jokes that day.) I took it to heart and was glad you wanted more from me than descriptions and appearance.

Toward the end of the session, when I talked about Sandy, my old friend who committed suicide, and my anger against parents who don't listen to psychiatrists unless something specific is prescribed, I was feeling anger without being aware of it. When it was over I felt I was getting sad and quiet and open. I felt a mild sensation, like pleasant nerves in a child dreaming of sex.

Then you commented that the session was over. Whenever I sense that cue, I begin to feel tentative again. The light that has been shining on me is about to go out. The psychiatrist's clumsy parliamentary procedure to get the patient gone. "And would two o'clock be all right?" you asked, which it wasn't, but I couldn't think firsthand. Only while going home did I have time to gnaw at that problem and make it into a big production number of possibilities.

At the time I decided I wouldn't try hard to write up these sessions, that I would let the style develop as my perceptions and experiences did. I gave up before I started writing this. I felt at the session like an exhausted person who has been reading and reading because of habit, who has stared only at the hard structure of print and not at the flight of words. Yesterday, like almost always, I was so self-conscious, glued to my surface, superficial structure of what I must say, what I must be. Reciting into a mirror. One mirror that wouldn't be bad luck if it were broken. (But those aren't fighting words. Just more yap.)

You said you wanted to hear only what happened in our sessions. At first that seemed limiting and then refreshing, because that cuts away the overhang of dense foliage. And you wouldn't read it for six months, which means that the sessions won't be a writing critique and there'll be no redeeming through words. And then later it dawned on me you had said "six" months, which was a comforting six months' guarantee.

October 14

DR. YALOM

THE SESSION was scheduled for 12:30. I saw Ginny in the waiting room at 12:25. I had something in my hand I wanted to give to my secretary, but it really wasn't important and I could have seen Ginny at 12:25. As things worked out, I screwed around with something relatively unnecessary and ended up taking her three minutes late. I can't understand why I do this with patients. Sometimes, no doubt, it is a measure of my own countertransference and resistance. But not with Ginny, I enjoy seeing her.

She looked well today, with a neat skirt, blouse and tights, and her hair almost brushed, but she was clearly very shaky and tremulous. For the first twenty to twenty-five minutes of the session we floundered without my knowing where the main thrust of the hour should go. It turned out that she had an extremely bad time of it last night, with waves of anxiety coming every ten to fifteen minutes, and these tightly bound to past terrible feelings and experiences, which seem to be the only things that give her a sense of continuity and time.

I first fiddled around with the timing of her night anxiety spells, wondering whether they were related to our sessions. There were three last week—one occurred the night before and one after our last hour, but the third one was somewhere in the middle of the week: so that didn't take us very far. Dealing with the ideational content of her anxiety spell was like walking on quicksand. I stepped in too deeply, was sucked down, and spent most of the hour trying to scramble out again, because it's all primitive, early, boundless material.

The next thing I tried was a happier choice. I simply became concrete and precise. I said, "Let's start from the beginning and really track down your day yesterday and what happened last night." I do this often with patients and advise my students to try out this approach, since it rarely fails to provide some foothold out of the mire of confusion. Well, Ginny went over her day—she had gotten up feeling pretty good and wrote for an hour or two. Although she tried

7

to minimize her writing, she admitted that she had been more active than usual, working presently on a novel. This makes me feel good; I take special pride, too much pride, in her being able to work at writing. Then she lay on her bed reading a book about female impotence written by a woman psychiatrist, whom I don't know, and becoming inundated with sexual feelings, she masturbated. And that was the beginning of her downfall for the day. Shortly afterwards she went out to the post office, accidentally meeting Karl, and was overcome with bad shameful, guilt feelings. Here she began to reproach herself in characteristic fashion; if she hadn't masturbated she could have saved it for Karl that night or maybe she could have gotten him sexually right then, etc., etc. Things went from bad to worse—the meal she cooked was a failure; at night when she was full of energy and wanted to go out, Karl was tired and went to bed; she wanted him to make love to her, but he fell asleep; she worried that maybe he was really rejecting her since he hasn't made love for two or three nights. She can't bring herself to try and approach him.

She also talked about last Saturday when Karl had been busy with people all morning and had walked by himself the rest of the day, not coming home until 8:30 at night, at which point she couldn't even say that she would like to walk with him sometimes. She just cried every time he came near her. I began to wonder about her ambivalent feelings towards him especially when she described her recurring fantasy that he would leave her and that she would go to Italy with her friend Eve, and write and drink chocolate. Well, all these things together made me think that despite her pledges of selfless allegiance to Karl, there's a part of Ginny that wants to tear loose from him. But it wasn't easy to pursue this; perhaps this is something Ginny is unable to deal with right now. Maybe not—I must not let her "fragile flower" pose control me to a point of impotent gentleness.

What I did do was to flood the room with Viktor Frankl. Now it happens that I had been reading one of his books last night and thinking about him. It always makes me disgusted with myself to read someone and then find myself using his techniques in my next therapy session. Be that as it may, I approached her as I think Frankl might have approached her, and I think I did rather well. The first thing I suggested to Ginny is the notion that she was born with anxiety, that her mother and father are anxious, and that it is not inconceivable to think she actually has a genetic source of anxiety, and perhaps even of sexual tension. I had a couple of things in mind. If Ginny has enough faith in me by now, I could help remove some of her guilt about masturbation, and on several occasions during the interview I went back again to the subject of masturbation, wondering what on earth she felt so guilty about. When she said things like, "it's weird" and "it's dirty" and that she should be "saving it for Karl," I told her that what was really weird was her vomiting every morning because some bio-energetic psychiatrist in the East had told her to do this as a means of relieving tension! I told her I saw nothing wrong with masturbating; if she has an excess of sexual tension, why not masturbate every day? This will not necessarily take away something from her sex relations with Karl, but might actually add to them, since she won't be so anxious. I was actually trying to do two things: symptom prescribing and relieving anxiety. I think it's going to be quite helpful, although I'm sure she'll go on to another type of symptom and concern.

The next thing I did was to point out to her that an inborn excess of anxiety and sexual tension (which I described in rather specific terms, i.e., an inability to metabolize adrenalin properly) is really not her core. She, Ginny, is something much more than these extrinsic factors. I guess I was getting into an examination of basic values. I asked her what it is in life that is really important to her, what she really values, what she can stand for. I was tempted to ask what types of things she would be willing to die for, but fortunately refrained. Well, she said some of the "right" things, to my point of view. She said she really wanted to get "into the light," "into the mainstream;" she deeply treasures her experience with Karl, and she ended by saying that her writing is very important. Naturally, like a reflex, I pounced on this, at which point she immediately called her writing "frivolous," adding that she knew I would say it wasn't. I followed suit and said, "It isn't frivolous." She laughed. I continued with the comments that no one else can do her writing for her, that it is something she alone can do, and that it's important, even if no one else ever reads it. She seemed to buy that, and that was about the end of the hour. I was being somewhat authoritarian, but I think that I've got to be with Ginny. I like her very much. I want to help her very badly. It's hard to believe sometimes that a poor tragic lilting little soul like this really exists and suffers so much.

October 14

GINNY

THE SESSION was very important for me. I think I managed to talk and think and feel through my tears. Not just cry and be done with it. I could keep more to the point, and not let sarcasm or charm get the upper hand. I reached a kind of balance.

I didn't use the therapy to take away my feelings. I felt less strained at the end. I still appreciate that you talk and tell me things. I don't feel like I'm in the room alone. If I were, I'd get confused and wander. When you said that all people masturbate, I burnt with shame because I thought you might be telling me something about yourself. I couldn't look at you. I pretend that everyone is structured and you can't see people's lives in private, only mine, which is transparent.

I think the session helped me use the tension I had and have to some good use and understanding.

I wonder why I always seem to place my men in a bad light, though. In retelling incidents, I know you get a one-sided view. It troubles me that I'm unfair and somehow I'll be punished.

I make it seem that Karl and I are like a frog and its insect in a school aquarium—so tight; when actually there's a lot more loose, good time between us than I let on. I guess I concentrate on the bad times because they are so annihilating.

As far as abstaining goes, I live by that. "I won't do this and maybe that will happen." I sort of have a checking account in my head, where I always have to be in debt to come out ahead.

After the session I felt centered; less awkward. I could give in to at least three impulses—to eat, to sit in the cactus grove near Stanford's grave, and to take deep breaths of the plants and trees.

When you told me I looked better, I felt bad that I didn't tell you how nice you looked in your landscape conglomeration of russet suit and various colored stripes coming from everywhere like rain. I withhold things.

Now whether I'll try the things you told me, I don't know. I know they'll depress me at first and punish me temporarily. And they'll depress me because they are happening in *my* life, with me privately. That's the reason abandonment scares me so much. I'm afraid of being abandoned by other people, since I long ago abandoned myself. So there's no *one* there when I'm alone. I am so camouflaged by my experience and you are asking me to accept some part of myself (nervousness) and go on from there.

October 21

DR. YALOM

BETTER TODAY. What was better? I was better. In fact I was very good today. It's almost as though I am performing in front of an audience. The audience that will read this. No, I guess that isn't completely true—now I'm doing the very thing I accuse Ginny of doing, which is to negate the positive aspects of myself. I was being good for Ginny today. I worked hard and I helped her get at some things, although I wonder if I wasn't just trying to impress her, trying to make her fall in love with me. Good Lòrd! Will I never be free of that? No it's still there, I have to keep an eye on it—the third eye, the third ear. What do I want her to love me for? It's not sexual —Ginny doesn't stir sexual feelings in me—no that's not completely true—she does, but that's not really important. Is it that I want to be known by Ginny as the person who cultivated her talent? There is some of that. At one point I caught myself hoping that she would notice that some of the books in my bookcases were nonpsychiatric ones, O'Neill plays, Dostoevsky. Christ, what a cross to bear! The ludicrousness of it. Here I am trying to help Ginny with survival problems and I'm still burdened down with my own petty vanities.

Think of Ginny—how was she? Pretty sloppy today. Her hair uncombed, not even a straight part, worn-out jeans, shirt patched in a couple of places. She started off by telling me what a bad night she had had last week when she was unable to achieve orgasm, and then couldn't sleep the entire night because she feared rejection from Karl. And then she started to go back to the image of herself as the same body of a little girl who used to lie awake all night when she

11

was in junior high school, hearing the same bird crying at three in the morning, and suddenly there I was again with Ginny, back in a hazy, clouded, mystical magical world. How fetching it all is, how much I would like to stroll around in that pleasant mist for awhile, but . . . contraindicated. That would really be selfish of me. So, I tackled the problem. We went back to the sexual act with her boyfriend and talked about some obvious factors that prevent her from reaching orgasm. For example, there are some clear things that Karl could do to help arouse her to reach climax, but she is unable to ask him, and then we went into her inability to ask. It was all so obvious that I almost feel Ginny was doing it on purpose to allow me to demonstrate how perceptive and helpful I can be.

So, too, with the next problem. She described how she had met two friends on the street and how she had made, as usual, a fool of herself. I analyzed that with her, and we got into some areas that perhaps Ginny hadn't quite expected. She behaved with them in a chance meeting on the street in such a way, she says, as to leave them walking away saying, "Poor pathetic Ginny." So I asked, "What could you have said that would have made them feel you were rather hearty?" In fact, I proved to her there were some constructive things she could have mentioned. She's trying out for an improvisational acting group, she has done some writing, she has a boyfriend, she spent an interesting summer in the country, but she can never say anything positive about herself since it would. not call forth the response, "Poor pathetic Ginny," and there is a strong part of her that wants just that reaction.

She does the same thing with me in the session, as I pointed out to her. For example, she had never really conveyed to me the fact that she is good enough to work with a professional acting troupe. Her self-effacing behavior is a pretty pervasive theme, going back to her behavior in the group. I shocked her a bit by telling her that she looked intentionally like a slob, that some day I'd like to see her looking nice, even to the extent of putting a comb through her hair. I tried to de-reflect her self-indulgent inner gaze by suggesting that maybe her core isn't in the midst of her vast inner emptiness, that maybe her core is as much outside of herself, even with other people. I also pointed out to her that although it is necessary for her to look inside to write, sheer introspection without writing or some other form of creation is often a barren exercise. She did say that she has done considerably more writing during the last week. That makes me very happy. It may be that she is just giving me a gift, something to keep me anticipating improvement.

I tried to get her to discuss her notion of my expectations for her, since this is a genuine blind spot for me. I suspect I have great expectations for Ginny; am I really exploiting her writing talent so that she will produce something for me? How much of my asking her to write instead of paying is sheer altruism? How much is selfish? I want to keep urging her to talk about what she thinks I'm expecting of her; I must keep this in focus—the Almighty God "Countertransference"—the more I worship it the less I give to Ginny. What I must not do is try to fill her sense of inner void with my own Pygmalion expectations.

She's a fetching, likeable soul, Ginny is. Though a doctor's dilemma. The more I like her as she is, the harder it will be for her to change; yet for change to occur, I have to show her that I like her, and at the same time convey the message that I also want her to change.

October 21

GINNY

(handed in three weeks later)

SOMETHING might happen if I were more natural looking. So I left my glasses on. Something might not happen though.

I spoke about that bad Tuesday night which turned out to have had a bad Tuesday beginning. The idea of a hearty, robust me, which you suggested and asked for, was very encouraging. My usual register of "success" is how much I have been released and done difficult things, like crying or thinking straight without fantasizing. And you pushed me in that direction.

I had fun at the session and before that could disturb me I

enjoyed the sensation, the buoyancy. I seemed to see alternatives to my way of acting. This lasted even when I went on the
campus afterwards. Though during the session and later I was
obviously questioning this optimistic feeling. Surely happiness
must be harder? Could I end it as a hearty wench?

I was looking at your way of treating me, like an adult. I wonder if you think I am pathetic or, if not, a hypocrite, or just an
old magazine that you read in a doctor's office. Your methods are
very comforting and absurd. You still seem to think that you can
ask me questions that I will answer helpfully or with insight. You
treat me with interest.

I think during the session that I am bragging, trying to show
myself off good. I am dropping little self-indulgent hints and
facts, like me being pretty (a real static fact), like the acting
group, like the good sentence I wrote (treading water in front
of your face). I know these are a waste of time since they don't
do me any good and are things that go through my head every
day with or without you. Even when you say, "I don't quite understand," that is a kind of flattery to my worst old habits of being
elusive in word and deed. And inside me I don't understand
either. God knows I know the difference between the things I say
and the things I feel. And my sayings are not satisfying most
times. The few times in therapy when I react in a fashion not
predestined by my mind, I feel alive in an eternal way.

So yesterday's experience was strange. I usually distrust the
things that are said. Parent pep talk. I give it to myself regularly.

But I didn't feel down when the session was over, or let down.
It was funny to hear you talk about my hair and dress. Kind of
like my father but not quite. Of course maybe you think Franny *
dressed good. To me she looked attractive but always seemed an
arm's length away. I look like a badly bent hanger with the
clothes slipping off. I like to look heroic, like I've just done
something. Though I wish I didn't have such an uncanny burlesque instinct in dressing. Sometimes I try and still look
schleppy.

The night after the session I couldn't sleep at all. There was
such a rush of blood in my chest and stomach and I could feel

---

* Group member.

my heart beating all night. Was it because there was no release in the session or that I couldn't wait for a new day to begin? I was raring to go. I am saying this now cause I don't want to say it in the next session.

I think it is wrong in therapy for me to be too self-conscious, to say things like, "I am feeling something in my leg." Those are probably cheap asides left over from sensory awareness afternoons, that stop the direction you are heading me in. You must get sick of them, infliction, indulgence.

It was funny when you said I couldn't make a career out of schizophrenia. (I still think catatonia is right up my sleeve.) In a sense this takes away a lot of the romance I have been flirting with. I feel awkward and lacking and can't connect in social situations. There must be another way. With Dr. M. ——— *
I think he thought the things I said were "far-out," weird, and that they should be recorded for their nuances. I think you know they're shit. I was always watching him write down things. I'm not aware of your face too much except that it seems to be sitting over there waiting for something. And you seem to have a lot of patience. I don't like to look at your face cause I know I haven't said anything. If it did light up at the wrong places, I'd begin to distrust you.

In these first few sessions I think I can be as bad as I want, so later the transition will seem lovely.

November 4

DR. YALOM

A FAINT metallic taste in my mouth after the interview. Not totally satisfied. Subdued, that's the word for it. Ginny came in apologizing for not having her description of the previous week's meeting.

---

* Group co-therapist.

She said that she had written it but hadn't typed it up the night before. When I questioned her more specifically, she said she was going to type it, but it had so many embarrassing things concerning masturbation that she didn't want to type it around Karl. I asked her whether she usually waits so long to type up what she's written. She said no, she usually does it the next day or two, but she knew she wasn't going to see me for two weeks. All the while, of course, I'm wondering what it meant to her not to have seen me last week, how much resentment or disappointment there was. It does seem odd that she has had a two-week interval and brings in no write-up, whereas previously she never failed to prepare her report. I am sure that at some level she is pouting and attempting to punish me.

Then the next thing she says tends to confirm my suspicions. She had seen me on Union Street in San Francisco with a woman. I said that was my wife, which she seems to have taken for granted; she added that the woman looked so young and pretty and that we seemed so happy together and that she (Ginny) had a good feeling about it. She also wondered whether that was the reason I hadn't seen her last week—whether I had just simply decided to spend the week with my wife. How did she feel about that? "Very good." I had my doubts!

I asked her whether or not she changes what she writes when she types it up. She states that she does sometimes. For example, the previous week she took out something that sounded like active flirtation with me because she was subsequently embarrassed at having written it. So the whole first part of the session was a subdued, even embarrassed interchange. I asked her at one point quite frankly whether or not she could discuss the subterranean part of the session, thinking that we could get at her unstated feelings. But she refused to nibble, and instead insisted that there really was nothing else she hadn't talked about. Things have gone so well, relatively speaking, that she can't specify a single problem.

And indeed they seem to have gone well; the waking up at night with terror seems to have subsided; she took the pill I gave her after the last session, which broke the cycle, although she was careful to let me know the pill wasn't entirely successful, since she had a real drowsy depressed hangover following it. To tell the truth, I forgot to write down exactly what medication I had given her: I remember only that it was a very mild tranquilizer, which should not have produced such strong sedative effects. But she has been writing, she has been active. She started to reel off a list of activities: German lessons twice a week, yoga, giving several dinner parties, dancing class. It does seem that she has been making some real strides. She is also grateful to me for having talked to her about masturbation; since that discussion she had had a sense of liberation and masturbated without feeling guilty or without fixating on the subject the rest of the day.

I was really impressed with how pretty she looked today. I have the chairs at a Sullivanian ninety degree angle and was looking at her more in profile. There have been times before, especially in the group, when I considered Ginny rather homely, and yet today I saw her as quite lovely.

Almost desperately attempting to provide me with an offering, she volunteered a couple of dreams. We languished in them for a few minutes, one of them presenting some pretty clear Oedipal components: a dream in which she was lying in bed and a man came in with a silver cigar for a penis. The associations to this had to do with her lying awake at night when she was young, listening to the sounds of a mattress squeaking which meant that her parents were having intercourse, and then an episode when she was twenty-one when she hurt her father by saying that her mother had once told her that sex wasn't always everything in life. There is abundant evidence of a desire to split her parents, to get between them, but it's folly for me to get into this with Ginny. Reconstruction of the past, interpretations, clarifications of this sort are not going to be helpful for Ginny. Visiting the past with her is a beguiling, charming voyage; but she knows the terrain far too well—it never fails to transport her away from today and from the benefit which I know will come from our understanding everything that happens between the two of us. So I switched the subject to the present.

She has been preoccupied with the fantasy that Karl will leave her, whereupon she'll go into a cabin in the woods and gradually become more mature. She exclaimed that this is horrible because it must mean that she wants Karl to leave her, but I pointed out that the fantasy has some redeeming features in that it is life-oriented and does offer the hope that she won't be extinguished if Karl were to leave. I used some paradoxical intention by suggesting that she deliberately force this fantasy to appear whenever Karl comes home late, and give it at

17

least five minutes' trial. The same thing with sexual relations: she states that she hears this little voice inside of her telling her that she's not really there, that she's separate, not really joined to Karl, that "this really isn't it," and then at the end of the act, it chastizes her for not having experienced enough. I suggested that she actively take the part of this voice, call it up as it were, in order to control it so that it doesn't control her. I do this in the hope that she will eventually see that it's nothing that happens to her, but it's something that she causes to happen.

Toward the end of the session she quoted something from Alexander Pope about a woman who seems similar to herself and she doesn't want to be like that. Having not read Pope for fifteen or twenty years, I found myself wishing that she would mention writers I'm more familiar with so I could have responded with more savvy and more ease. I think this also reflects some feelings of tension that I have about tomorrow's presentation at the Modern Thought seminar where my interest in literature is vastly exceeded by glaring gaps in knowledge.

November 4

GINNY

I WAS pretty nervous yesterday. I just grabbed at straws, thinking of something to say, that's how seeing you that day with your wife came up. I was inside the car with Eve discussing *The Freedom of Sexual Surrender*, a book which discredits clitoral orgasm as something that doesn't happen in a mature woman's body. So in the middle of this sexual talk, you and your wife crossed the crosswalk in front of us, like a stunt in a T.V. comedy.

I saw that what I do is pretend that some part of me is doing what actually I am doing. For instance, the last five minutes, that "part of me" happened to look at your open pants and imagine that I saw something. I was immediately embarrassed, and started talking about something different. You immediately crossed your legs. And I had divided myself because I had done something that "I," as I am known, don't do. And I goad myself into it because I know it breaks my concentration and progress. It's like doodling with your mind.

I always like it when you give me directives. I become much more aware of my behavior, not as something magical, but just as behavior. Last night I became aware of how the fear starts. I think of something, I hold my breath to listen, that hurts my stomach, makes me feel like I'm in an elevator and can't get off. And before I know it, I'm on an unlucky floor.

The session made me very nervous, more nervous than when I went in.

November 12

DR. YALOM

AN ODD sort of session. I didn't think I'd be much good for anything since I had only two hours sleep last night. I stayed at a friend's home on the ocean, and the strangeness of sleeping outside and the pounding of the waves had kept me up all night. I thought then how ironic it was that I should be seeing Ginny the next day since she has often come in with complaints of being unable to sleep. My being awake last night was different in that it was a comfortable state of wakefulness and I enjoyed watching and hearing the ocean and reading Kazantzakis, but I've had those other kinds of night too. Never do I feel more like a fraud than when after a sleepless, anxious night I counsel some poor insomniac who in truth slept more hours than I. But who would follow a general who on the eve of battle walked around wringing his hands? I didn't cancel the hour because I felt functional today and during the session was hardly aware of my state of fatigue.

I was approximately ten minutes late, though, and to help stay awake brought a cup of coffee into my office, which is unusual. I did offer her one, which she refused with embarrassment. She began by talking about her envy of her younger sister, who is now visiting. She sees her sister as so much more decisive, more "committed" than she, for example, in choosing to live with someone. I tried to help her understand the fact that this is only an attitudinal posture; I asked her whether or not it meant that her sister really did have more of a sense of commitment and wondered with her whether it meant only that her sister could overlook some of the negative feelings she had about a situation, or perhaps even engage in self-deception about some of her conflicting feelings. What's to be envied about such "positiveness"? She heartily agreed that this was so.

I then went on to talk with her about the little imp inside that strips all pleasure from every one of her endeavors, stops her from enjoying sex, enjoying her trip to Europe, from enjoying life. This is it, her one and only life. No rainchecks, no replays when she is feeling better. "Ginny, you're going through life right now and can't postpone it till another time." I'm not sure how helpful that tact was. Wasn't I being overly pedantic?

The other major theme was her anger or rather her lack of anger in infuriating situations. For example, she talked about her relationship to her landlady who is so maddening, so flighty that she drives everyone crazy. Ginny's response to this woman is only to "feel more dead inside" and to make a greater effort to be nice to her. We worked on how a feeling of anger or annoyance toward the other person can somehow get converted into a sense of personal deadness. Later in the discussion I was afraid that she interpreted my comments as a suggestion *not* to be nice to people and to let all her angry feelings out, whereupon I reassured her that she shouldn't feel ashamed of being "nice" or generous—these are genuine traits which don't have to be reduced to something else, but it is necessary for her to understand her true feelings in these situations. She went on to say that when she engages in generous or altruistic acts, she always manages somehow to turn them into vices, and I in effect told her to stop this Freudian reductionism and accept generosity or gentleness as positive and important truths about herself which stand by themselves and don't require further analysis.

She doesn't talk much about her feelings toward me. She felt tense today and uneasy. Whenever I asked what she was feeling at a specific moment, she always came up with an abstract generalization about the course of her life, without dipping into the vast subterranean pool of emotions underlying each of our interviews. When I asked specifically about this, she said much that is unstated emerges when she reflects back upon the sessions while writing her reports. She mentioned several times in an offhand fashion that it takes much of the day to prepare herself for the meeting with me. She had a two-hour wait for a bus to get back to San Francisco so that it's really an entire day's affair, and she is very anxious lest she not use the time constructively. At the same time I think that the relationship between us is a very solid one. I find myself very peaceful and warm when I'm with Ginny. She's a remarkable person, remarkable not only in her capacity for anguish, but in her sensitivity and beauty.

November 19

DR. YALOM

GINNY dressed in patched jeans and appearing particularly Ginny-gentle and Ginny-fragile. Speaking softly, she confessed that she didn't have her write-up of last week—she hadn't written it till five days after our last session, hadn't typed it up yet, and there is even a possibility that she had lost it. I felt this was terribly important and that we were going to have to spend a great deal of time on the subject. She dug in her heels and wouldn't budge. She had no ideas or associations to the issue when I brought it up. I got a bit stronger each time around, stating, that, for example, it is highly unlikely that she should suddenly forget her assignment; why is it now that five days pass between her session and her review of it, whereas previously she wrote it the day after? When she responded that she is lazy, I pushed her further and asked why she is lazy *now*. But nothing came of my question. I felt strongly she wasn't going to be able to talk about anything else and so it was. She stumbled about trying to find some other issues, without success. At the very beginning of the session she had mentioned that she had gotten into a quarrel with Karl about psychiatrists, since he thinks psychiatrists are really unnecessary and unhelpful. I wondered aloud whether or not she was feeling that she had to choose between Karl and me. This too got nowhere. A bit impatient with her, I let her wallow in her helplessness for awhile.

Perhaps the turning point, as I look back on it, appeared when I said cryptically, "There is no magic after all." Ginny asked what I meant, but I knew she knew, and she agreed that she knew even after she asked the question. I meant that there was no magic after all in my taking her out of the group and seeing her individually, that nothing was really going to happen until she made something happen. She felt a little alarmed at that and wondered whether I took her out of the group on purpose in order to show her that there was no hope for her outside of herself. I assured her, of course, that this wasn't the case, but that there is indeed no hope for her unless she moves from within.

For the rest of the interview I tried to push her more and more into a discussion of her and me. At one point she said that I looked something like a man she had recently seen in a film who was an old letch. When I asked about sexual feelings she may have had toward me, I received no leads. I then began asking her how she wanted me to see her, how much she had to screen her statements because of what she expected I would feel about them. She stated that she only wanted me to know she was trying to get well. But wasn't she nonetheless deceiving both of us, since she admitted that she wasn't trying much of the time?

Only later on in the interview was she able to talk about wanting to be a woman in front of me (as she sat there like a child), that she wanted to appear attractive to me, yet nevertheless she wore these dungarees today because she wasn't feeling well last night and wanted to sleep on the bus. (She had a migraine headache last night, the second migraine immediately prior to a visit with me). I was quite rough with her today. For example, I made it clear that although she says she wants to please me, she deliberately did something designed to displease me, i.e., not bringing in the written material. I again pointed out, and this time it finally seemed to take, that there was something behind her not writing which was probably connected to her feelings toward me; it was striking that at the same time she stopped writing, she also stopped talking in the sessions. I also decided to help her test reality by pointing out that writing a summary of the previous interview is not optional—that's part of an adult (thought I didn't use this word) contract she has made. What was unstated was the implicit threat, which I am perfectly serious about, that I will not see her without her keeping this part of the contract. She seemed a bit subdued by this, said she felt like a young student in front of a substitute teacher.

Later when discussing her attractiveness as a woman, she expressed some bad feelings about her body, especially about her elongated labia, which makes her feel ugly and unlike a woman. I suspect this is the analogue of men feeling they have penises which are small. Since she has never, in fact, compared this area of her body with anyone else's and secretly uses this to feed her negative image of herself, I jestingly asked her who she's ever checked it out with.

Then I asked if she felt she was now pleasing me more. She said that she was. I asked her when it began. She started to cry, uttering through the tears that it was as though she had to talk about unpleasant parts of herself to please me and herself. That wasn't the way I felt and told her so. I am pleased when she is simply more honest with her feelings and stops resisting and denying issues. It makes little difference to me whether or not these are intrinsically unpleasant or pleasant subjects as long as she's being honest. She seemed to hear that, and we ended up on a closer and more harmonious note, I think, though the hour was an unsettling one for her. I tried to reassure her somewhat by reminding her that next Wednesday is the day before Thanksgiving, but that I will be here if she is planning to come. I guess what I was really saying is, "I do care about you and I'll be here, even though it's practically a holiday."

November 19

GINNY

AS I was coming up on the bus I said "unfocused" and that became the cue word for the morning. Three-fourths of the session that's how I felt. So as not to appear stupid or boring I had to concentrate on what I was doing. Even though you are seeing it simultaneously I have to say things like "I'm talking into my nails, mumbling." I have to say things inside me first. Kind of sharing the observation with you so as not to leave you out completely. The part I brought you of me doesn't really touch deeply, even though I can mumble about it for forty minutes. It is like going to the zoo and looking at an animal but really only focusing on the cage. You can't see the animal for the cage.

As for telling you that you looked like Don Lopez of *Tristana,* I said that to Karl first as a kind of crack joke about you. Having fun at your expense. But it really wasn't a bad thing in my eyes. I would like to be able to induce such a dream where you could take an active role.

I first started feeling real in the session when I said I felt sad because I knew I was disappointing you. I never felt like I was disappointing you in the group since I didn't think you were expecting anything in particular. There were so many other mute faces. You seemed more imaginary than you do now. Then I started talking, saying things that could either be put in the "sexual category" or the "bad things." But as I was saying them I saw that I was bundled up inside this wrapping, these leggings, this smile of a little girl. I think it's always when I feel this presence inside me that I start to cry. I feel like I have to drag this pitiful, but real, kid around in me. And the most important question was when you asked me, "Do you think of yourself as a woman?" I knew, "No, no." That's why there's always a certain amount of gameiness and flirtation, but it is more me flirting with a woman's identity. I can't really be violated. Not a woman seduced by a man. The landlady and I in our fights are not two women. It's a crank and a little girl who has done something wrong and wants to get on the good side of life.

Then you said, "Have you pleased me?" I knew I had but when we started analyzing it, that brought the other part of me back, that unreal equal I feel I have to be. I just want to be bundled up and rocked by you. I think I got off the track. That's when I agreed with the categories. I hate to look back over my shoulder like that and I always do. You ask for it. You prompt me into analyzing sensations, whereas I just want to have them.

But before, while I was talking, I had pleasurable feelings. A relief to talk, not to have to keep up such a face. Of course my melodramatic, sarcastic agent was booking me up on the sideline, with the title "Queer." Kind of to taunt me out of my feelings and to change the subject.

So then I said, "It will be so awful, the thoughts that will come out." I didn't mean that I was trying to pacify and agree with the sarcastic part. Actually I felt grateful. It didn't seem like facts I was telling, just feelings.

I also felt a progression. Like I didn't want to start from nothing next session. Didn't want to end the session, either.

That dream of the pulled flesh was one of the rare sexual dreams where flesh is actually involved. The people around me who were pulling my flesh down were doctors. I concentrated on the session for the forty minutes after, when I sat on the grass and wrote this. But after that I did practical things that I thought might help me. I was aware of pleasurable thoughts this week, moments with Karl that seemed real without tears. Also, I was aware of that feeling that is not a feeling, but a suspension. Like before I know I have to write and don't, before I know I have to type this and don't, before I know I should be thinking of this and don't. That a great part of my time is spent in holding back. Just like I do in the session, an imperfect replica of life.

November 25

DR. YALOM

A FLUID and close encounter with Ginny today. It should have been bad but I worked hard and well, and Ginny was willing to stretch herself. A migraine headache, she says; it started yesterday. Another one, I said. I think that's several occurring the day before seeing me, and also those night panics the day before our sessions. I inquire about this, gently of course. She plays dumb. I ask again, in fact I ask several times. She plays very elusive, she doesn't know what I mean. She answers each of my questions concerning her feeling about seeing me without using the pronoun "you." This makes me even more convinced that she's avoiding me. I'm surprised. We know each other so well, now, it's been two years, and it surprises me to rediscover that she still can't talk about me and even has to evade thinking about me. She comes up with the reason that if she talks about me, this will make it even harder for her to relate to Karl. That's magic, I think, and say so, as if giving voice to thoughts makes them a reality. She nods and talks a bit more. I bluntly comment upon her inability to address me as "you" and wonder about my role in her fantasies. There, she stretches a bit and gently opens the door. She reveals that she has had a fantasy of writing a story, earning $300 for it and buying me a gift. I try to push her into the fantasy, asking what the gift was. She can't remember. I ask her why she wanted to give me a gift. She says, to repay my faith in her. Therefore, it had to be in writing a story. I wonder what else it means to her to give me a gift.

At this point I am coyly inviting her to say something loving. She can't. She says it reminds her of having given a gift to a teacher, but you usually give a teacher a present only at the end of term. I become braver and wonder aloud, "Isn't it possible to give a teacher a gift because you like him?" At this point she makes the connection and says disarmingly, "Well, you know I like you." I maintain my composure: "You say that so easily now!" I remind her that she has eschewed that admission ever since we have known each other. Moreover, liking is not undimensional—liking me must have a considerable number of facets, and yet she cannot express any of them. She listens. She opens up a bit more and talks about how she liked me last year when I was leading the group and how she would silently cheer for me, if I were to say something that would help some of the other patients, only this year it's different because she is the patient and it's hard to be subject and observer at the same time. Silence. I ask her where her thoughts are. She flits away and says she had started to think about her old boyfriend, Pete. I let her go.

We talked about Pete and she tells me how he had just called her minutes before Karl walked through the door, how she told Pete she had to hang up and then felt guilty for it and called him back in twenty minutes and was obsessed with all the bad things that she had done. I went over each of the bad things, as I have in the past with other events, indicating to her on each occassion how she hyper-analyzes. Why can't she stop sometimes with a sheer good feeling or sense of altruism without always turning it into a vice? In fact she did care about Pete, she gave him what she could, she was happy the next day when she learned that he had made a new girlfriend. In each case she turns it against herself by saying that she didn't care *enough* or that she didn't give *enough*, or it was for her own interest that she tried to do something fine for him. The self-destructive alchemist inside of her changes everything from good to evil. I tried to underscore this by pointing out that she has been rather magnanimous in her feelings toward him, and, of course, I stumbled, as I always do, over the word "magnanimous!" She responded by stumbling over the word "fecund," which was the last thing she said: "It will be a fecund week." We moved today, as we usually do, when I can open her up about her feelings toward me.

November 25

GINNY

THE THING about a migraine is you can't have anything ruffle your balance. That is the posture I've taken in sessions. Inside I think I want myself to be changed radically—no vestige or shred or smile to remain. So when you try to salvage some of my ways of doing things, showing they're not all bad, it's sort of comforting. But the remnant doesn't mean too much. I feel sarcastic about your praise.

When I used to be religious, God was a kind of catalyst between me and my relations with the world. I would give up so much for things to go good in the outside world. In this way I bargained off years of life, said I wouldn't care if I never had a boyfriend and never got married, so long as my parents would stay alive. I, on my part, was never as good as I promised, but in the sloppy interchange between me and God, things worked out on His part, even though I fell short.

EVERY DAY GETS A LITTLE CLOSER

I would do anything just to keep myself in a relationship. Even though I might be totally camouflaged, so the other person doesn't know I'm there.

That's what I do with you, I think. Try to measure up, but I don't want to disturb you or myself. And I know I'm not supposed to entertain you—so somewhere in between I sit. I am sort of sustaining the exhibit, not smashing it or finishing it.

When I talked about Pete and you said, "Why do you have to get to the bad side?" That's like saying that a person would be pretty if her nose hadn't grown that extra inch. If I try deliberately stopping after a single thought before it becomes fetid and heavy, I'd be aware that I was doing it. Vicious circles are my natural train of thought.

I know I want too much attention, undivided attention. But just a physical proximity, not too much in-depth attention.

I am very on guard in session now. I know you want me to probe my feelings toward you, and because they are not just bubbling out of my mind and face, I feel silly digging for them. I have always been honest, I thought, in saying what I am thinking, but all I've really been is the top part of the flower, and never crawled under the dirt and exposed roots. My sincerity is pretty and probably superficial.

I feel in everything I must hold back, and when I do it, as my emotions and me are receding from view (it inevitably leads to that) I am the first to censure.

And there are so many words of censure, I watch my actions, justify them. I see that I am not rewarded. And that is right.

These words don't pertain to any particular incident. They are just a view that I am stuck with. It's why I sometimes can't concentrate on particular incidents.

December 2

DR. YALOM

I FELT very alert, eager to see Ginny, eager to make contact with her today. She came in and handed me what she had written from last week. As I put it down on the desk, I saw her eyes watching me. She looked as though she were feeling something, and I said to her, "Go ahead and say it." She couldn't say it. She said there was nothing. Then she said that she had just rewritten the report this morning because it was all in scraps of paper. I asked her how long she had taken to write it. She said she had spent about a half hour on it, but then hastily added, "That's all I spend on anything." I wondered whether this was an apology. She denied that, saying she never spends more time writing anything, that she never thinks about what she writes, but that the words just flow from her.

The official start of the hour. A complaint. Things aren't good with Karl, sexually. Then she combined this grievance with another —it had been like this ever since I had given her those pills. She couldn't elaborate. I got the feeling that there was a not-so-hidden accusation against me in her statement, but no further traces of that were visible during the hour.

She had written well the day before: two good solid hours of work producing ten pages, but then she felt so sloppy and bad inside the rest of the day. I spent a while trying to investigate that statement, wondering if we could rationally reexamine her feelings. She could immediately see the fallacy of her value judgment. I asked her what she meant by "sloppy?" My theory was that she at least spends the rest of the day generating ideas for the next morning's writing, so that anything she did the rest of the day could be construed as useful. She wouldn't accept that, insisting that mornings and afternoons are completely compartmentalized—nothing feeds into the morning after except an occasional dream. Oh yes, there was a dream of a big woman with big breasts and a big penis, she was lying on top of this woman and that scared her a good bit. She mentioned the dream a couple of times. She wanted to work on it, I didn't. If I fall into Ginny's phantasmagorical dream world, I lose touch with the flesh and blood person, and we both lose touch with what's happening between the two of us, and it's on the thread of what's passing between us that I think everything depends. So I didn't bite at the dream-bait and instead returned to her feelings of sloppiness. From there we went into an endless cycle of her feeling sad, of her feeling that she lets everyone down, that nothing she has is worthwhile. It soon became clear, as I have said to her many times before, that all of her experiences are filtered through that background music of self-deprecation with the constant refrain, "I'm not worth anything, I don't deserve anything, I'm bad."

I tried another reasonable tact. How come, I wonder with her, many people like you, many people find something of value in you? Could it be that their judgment of you is better than yours? She doesn't answer, but I know what she is thinking. "They don't really know me; nobody can perceive the emptiness inside of me." She talks of her inability to continue anything. For example, she went through the motions of coming to the group, but was passive within it for a whole year. She only pretends to live and to give. She does the same with Karl. I wonder aloud why Karl chooses to spend his life with her. She undercuts herself again by claiming that she puts on a show for him.

Then I give her the loaded question. "Why do I see you? Why do I continue to see you?" She seems flustered and says she doesn't know, and is near tears. She talks about not being able to give me anything, that she desperately wants to be able to walk out of here improved, no longer desperate and hopeless. She doesn't know how to do it. I want to say to her that obviously I'm continuing to see her because I see something of value in her. I don't say that explicitly but it comes out implicitly. She says she can't even look at me. I ask her to look at me and she does and suddenly I become aware of the fact that she hasn't really looked at me for any length of time before. So we look at each other's eyes for awhile in the session today.

She says she suddenly feels dizzy and nauseated and very tense and then begins to weep. I try to find out what's behind the weeping. She can say only that she doesn't deserve to get any kind of warmth from me, and yet feels herself on the edge of receiving this warmth. She must do something first to deserve it. What has she got to give me? If I wanted her to clean up my office, she'd do it. (I recall how eagerly she told me about a series of novels written by Anthony Powell, an English writer, and how timidly she tried to suggest that I, she is sure, would enjoy these.) I commented again on her feelings of blackness and unworthiness. I label it a myth and wonder where the myth arose. She says it's not so much blackness or evil as emptiness. I tell her that she can't even look in my eyes without being filled with feeling, so that emptiness too is a myth. I hope that's true. Perhaps I'm not giving her profound feeling of schizoid emptiness its due. And yet I don't want to pay attention to that right now because she is filled with feeling, and I'd rather work on that level. She weeps when I say that. I reassure her that we are together through thick and thin and I'm going to see this out with her. She tries to trip off and starts to talk about the dream. I bring her back by saying that I think the dream must be of me, that I am the big person with breasts and a penis. She then ties me together with her female therapist in the East, who has big breasts.

Toward the end of the hour she feels the onset of a migraine. She states she was so proud of not having a headache before coming to see me this week, but the danger period is not over. I spend the last three minutes giving her some relaxation procedures, starting from the toes up, with the major suggestion that her eyeballs sink back into her head, since she complains that they are practically bulging out of her skull. The relaxation exercises seem to be helpful.

Ginny leaves feeling much better, and, ironically, it has stopped raining. Water had been flowing for much of the hour on both sides of the window. Ginny says it's as if she had been drinking something fattening and is suddenly filled up. Maybe that's true. I think of Madame Sechahaye * and symbolic realization. That's O.K. I can work with that too.

December 2

GINNY

WHEN I came in after a week that was fecund in the wrong direction I didn't expect anything, probably just to confess that much.

When I first started crying it was out of tension and frustration. But for once it didn't stay there. It didn't even jump immediately to release, as it sometimes does. Yesterday you broke

---

* Sechahaye, M., *Symbolic Realization* (N.Y.: International Press, 1951.)

the circle. You sort of guided me out. I felt that if ever I came in again, non-seeing and waiting and on-looking, pretending that there is nothing on my mind but drizzle, I'll just be acting coy.

Things seemed to change. I took new steps. I had been refusing to answer your repeated question, "What do I mean to you?" because I could only have answered with words. Because I insisted on limiting myself to words. Kind of like a short-answer quiz.

Even at the end when you told me to close my eyes and relax, other times I would have been impatient that time was going by, and that it wouldn't work. But something was happening. I didn't get a migraine, then or all day.

When I went to leave and the sun really had broken through, as though we were in a Hollywood psychological thriller, I said "Well, it will rain again." A soggy answer, I realized, a flip answer, but I didn't have to flaggelate myself for having given the wrong answer and failed somehow. I took it for the sarcastic habit it is. But because I felt different inside, I could quiet the mumbling. I didn't feel like a warehouse of echoes as I usually do.

All through the session it seemed I was trying to go back on my old track, to involve us in the old habits of dangling sentences. And you kept bringing me back.

Also, I was mostly aware, except at the end, that it's just me there and you. Not worrying that what I was doing would detract from other people—Karl, my parents, my friends.

When I felt dizzy and nauseous I tolerated it. I didn't immediately think of drinking three glasses of warm salted water and making myself vomit with my thumb. I try to feel some of the sensation on the other side of the nausea which is not mere fear, but actually pleasurable feelings.

I feel a little dizzy, aware now when I talk to people, how I do not make contact. With everyone I probably don't have to go through a procedure like yesterday's, but I wonder why with some people I choose to hide.

When you said I was tingling with emotions, flooded with them, it was so nice. The rest of the day I was aware of more feeling and sadnesses. But things were easier. I was not plugged with indecision. I felt clearer. Though the rest of the week I regressed and plummeted.

December 9

DR. YALOM

GINNY ebullient today. She used that word to describe something she wrote—a word I haven't used for years—it was right for her today. She was high-spirited, optimistic, somehow changed by last week's session. She came in saying she really wished we weren't meeting for a few more days because she is not "ready." That meant that she had such high hopes for today's session, but didn't see how she could get herself into the proper frame. She wasn't sure that she could do it today. I had to ask her what "it" was. So much has been happening to me this week, the last meeting was still a little sketchy. However, within a minute or two it suddenly burst into my mind, and I remembered everything that had happened. She said "it" was expressing her feelings clearly. Unimaginatively but doggedly I suggested that "it" was especially expressing feelings to me and about me.

She said her reason for not being ready was that she had had to prepare a surprise birthday party for Karl, which used up a lot of energy. That explanation made me more convinced than ever that, at some level, she was pitting me against Karl, that she could give only to either him or me. It was as though she had only a per- manently limited supply of love and affection and what she gave to one was taken from the other. When I expressed this to her, she remarked that when she came back from last week's session, she told Karl that I had said she was tingling with feeling. He scoffed at that and hugged her in a playful, mocking fashion. That was a curious business because I don't think I used the word "tingling"— it's not one of my words. She, too, was a bit confused and then changed the subject to sex and her present inability to have an

33

orgasm with Karl. Suddenly she stopped and said that I wasn't interested in what she was saying any more. This is an entirely new kind of comment from Ginny. She has rarely, in fact probably never, said something like that in the past. I wanted to encourage her for criticizing me and dealing with me so directly, but at the same time I had to tell her that she was wrong, because as a matter of fact I was listening with much interest. In fact, I had been on the verge of asking her what Karl could do to help her have an orgasm and what prevented her from telling him. Specifically I was wondering why she couldn't allow him to masturbate her. So I said both things: I assured her that she misread me and also implied that I was glad she raised the question. Later in the session I said so more explicitly.

Did I enter into her sexual life in some way? She replied she had been so optimistic the day after our last session, but the feeling had gradually disappeared and she had a migraine the following evening. I commented on her end-run around my question and repeated it. She then told me a recent dream in which she and Mr. Light were looking at each other for a long period of time. Mr. Light was a former teacher who had encouraged her writing and had apparently fallen in love with her. At their very last meeting he had put his hand under her tiny brassiere. A month later he visited her and her family and she spent a day with him at the beach, but had not made love with him, mainly because of lack of a suitable opportunity. Later he wrote her that he had been considering leaving his wife for her. I asked for associations to Mr. Light and she produced only, "I'll show you the light." I thought it was clear that Mr. Light in some way represented me—not only in my showing her the light but also in the fact that she and I had looked into each other's eyes last session much more than before. She then recalled another dream fragment of a rough cowboy, not Karl, but a boyfriend who reminds her of Karl, pulling her by the arms to get her away. She was obviously embarrassed while telling this story about Mr. Light and I asked her why. She said it was because she was handling something that was once very serious in a flippant, light-hearted way. My suspicion was that she was embarrassed because she was indirectly talking about me. I asked her whether or not the relaxation exercise I gave her at the end of the session was a type of sexual experience. She said it wasn't, but that it really made her feel good and she was glad for it. After the session she had gone to the ladies room and lay down on the couch and relaxed some more. She said she has tried various relaxing exercises in encounter groups, always with little success, so she had a negative feeling when I started. It was successful for it did thwart the migraine that day.

I pursued Mr. Light and asked her whether the idea of my leaving my wife had occurred to her. She said that she has seen my wife and that my wife appeared not too unlike herself, only a more integrated woman. My wife and I seem right for each other and she suspects a separation would not be likely. Mr. Light's wife, however, was a different kind of woman, fat and unintellectual, so that Ginny represented something really different to him.

I remarked that I was saying many unusual things today. She wondered whether they were genuine—or was I just testing her in some fashion? I told her the truth—I was saying things in a much more uncensored fashion than is usual for me. I could say almost the first thing that came to my mind, such as the questions about how I fit into her sexual life and what she thinks of me and my wife, because I felt her to be much more open and receptive and unafraid to look at me. (We did continue today to look at each other far more than we have in the past.)

During the session she recited a few lines of her poetry, especially from a satirical poem written in response to a speech by a woman's liberationist. I was much amused by some of the clever lines, e.g., "Do you want us to walk with breasts unfurled?" But then she began to chastise herself for having written this, calling it small and frivolous. I asked her if there's not a more generous descriptive word and she used ironic or witty. Irony comes hard for her; she finds it almost impossible to express feelings of disagreement or anger without subsequent self-castigation. She thinks she doesn't have the right to criticize; in fact she doesn't allow herself any rights at all, and that's still a big part of her being a little girl and having to keep the lid on any part of her not inconsiderable reservoir of anger.

She left the session, I think, somewhat disappointed because of unrealistically high expectations. Toward the end of the hour I felt a different kind of feeling settling in, and my hunch is that the high optimism will be dampened and she will be somewhat depressed as she recognizes some of her unrealistic feelings about me. That's not to say that I don't feel good about Ginny and that we aren't moving along together, but I'm aware that an extra, rather powerful bit of feeling has been placed on me, that has nothing to do with me and nothing to do with our relationship but rather with ghosts from the past.

December 9

GINNY

I THINK I was trying to entertain you. I wanted to go deeper than last week but when I came in I didn't feel in the mood. I just wanted to enjoy us.

All of last week didn't wear off, however, since I was more aware of you-me looking, at least. I pulled myself in that direction.

If you had scolded or said "What's this game you're playing this week?" I would have changed. Instead you didn't seem to mind (that I was a waitress and you were a client).

We did a good job of analyzing someone whose motives were there but not emotions.

I don't feel bad. I told most everything that happened to me that was important, but without a compelling center of a need to change.

I didn't see any of the parallels with Mr. Light until you made me see them. In a way that dream was showing and experiencing the meaningfulness and pleasure in my small relationship with him, and my telling it to you emphasized the absurd side. Maybe I told you the dream to show you the absurd ironic side to my looking you in the eyes. To put the last session in its ridiculous perspective (with the cement of sarcasm).

Actually the session was me in the purest, as I am every day. All the things I want to change. The sarcastic, giddy, anecdotal time-passing images. I feel angry in perspective that I carried on and enjoyed so this superficial side. The revenge is there's nothing to write in this write-up because there were no revelations. (Except maybe the intellectual idea that there's a parallel between you and Mr. Light and then the perennial loss that I did not explore that in the session; only named it and went over old stories out of my compulsive past.) Because I was talking very outside any emotional senses. No aftermath.

II

A Long Spring

(January 6–May 18)

DR. YALOM

REVISITING. We turn to the past. Three weeks ago Ginny called to tell me she had suddenly decided to go home for Christmas, since Karl and all of her friends were leaving and she couldn't bear the thought of being here alone. As she described her visit East, it sounded like a journey into guilt. She introduced it by saying that she should have stayed longer, that she was there only thirteen days, that she hadn't been fair to her mother or her father, that she spent only three days with them and the rest of the time with her friends and she hadn't been sensitive enough to her parents' needs. On Christmas day Mother had picked up and gone to the beach for three hours by herself because she was upset. Ginny came down, asked her father where Mother was, and said, "What's the matter with Mother—is she crazy, going out to the beach today?" Immediately Ginny's sister bombed her for her thoughtlessness in saying such a thing.

In a period of five to ten minutes, as Ginny was describing her home, I suddenly had an entirely new perspective on the making of Ginny. In so many ways I envisioned her mother as a guilt-inducing machine. When I expressed some of these thoughts to Ginny, which I did fairly openly, Ginny quickly rushed to her mother's defense: for example, Mother had gone to the beach "to experience some of her more stormy emotions." She then tried to shift the onus of blame to her domineering and matriarchal grandmother. I agreed that it wasn't her mother's intention to create guilt, but, nevertheless, that's what happened. Ginny continued by considering how awful it is for her mother because her two daughters are leaving her. I suggested that a mother's job is to prepare her children to be able to leave home, but Ginny brushed this aside almost impatiently.

Then she talked (in my language) about her inability to differentiate her ego boundaries from those of her mother. She said that her psychotherapist in New York was always shocked that she and her mother would use the bathroom at the same time. She wanted Mother to see her bras, she wanted to show her figure to

Mother and tell her how she too was growing fat and having the same type of body as her mother. She defended Mother by saying that she had made it possible for Ginny to transfer to a first-rate college, instead of staying on safe home ground. I reminded her, although I'm sure without effect, that things are much more subtle than that, that Mother probably has very mixed feelings about her living away and gives her two conflicting messages at the same time (ye old doublebind—classical form).

And so we talked about these things, though I suspect without much benefit for Ginny. (I persisted because it was illuminating to me; I gained a much clearer view of Ginny within her family context.) She wants so much for things to be different, had such hopes of going home and really breaking through. But what does she really want? She wants to return to a warm, loving idyllic childhood that never in fact existed. Or, at least I think it never existed. It's remarkable how little Ginny and I have talked about her childhood. I'm very wary of getting sucked into a Proustian recircling of the past. Stay in the future with Ginny. She'll have a different past soon.

She told me a dream, prefacing it and concluding it at least a half dozen times with the commentary that it was a silly dream that didn't mean anything. Naturally I see this as secondary revision and can only conclude that the dream was in fact very important. The dream was that I was having dinner with a number of gurus, who were obviously incompetent, and yet I was saying that they were O.K. The dream was unsettling because in it she said she ought to have someone new to work with. However, in her waking state she knew this wasn't so and thus decided to hide the dream from me, lest I take it seriously. Her associations to this were newspaper articles she had read about me (which had misquoted me somewhat), in which I criticized Esalen and other kinds of encounter groups, especially an encounter group leader who led a group that she had been in.

She talked about her new job as a traffic guard. She finds it very humiliating and then joked with me saying that I thought I was working with a writer and now I'm working with a policewoman. I became very uncomfortable at that and felt that I was in a sense, at least in her mind, doing the same thing her mother had been doing, making great demands on her for production, and she sensed that she had to be a writer and produce for me rather than for herself. I said as much to her, but with little effect. No doubt there is more than a little truth therein. I do want Ginny to be able to write. And no doubt in my fantasy I would be very pleased were she to become an exceedingly able writer. Yes, I can't deny that. However, it shouldn't make that much difference to me if that were never to occur, and if Ginny were to come out of her work with me having grown and having found some peace with herself and were never to write another word, that would be O.K. too. I hope the truth really is that I am seriously interested in Ginny as a person, and I'm having only a mild flirtation with Ginny, the writer.

January 6

GINNY

IF I WERE accused of a crime I would be my own best witness. Whenever I talk about people I love, I always make them seem guilty and I do this with a smile. Because if I'm guilty, they're guilty, guiltier in your eyes. I was giving you information, though I don't know why, because you're not going to make any evaluation or come up with an answer or plan. Anything good that happens in this therapy happens simultaneously.

I knew I was giving you ammunition against my parents. That made me feel worse. Especially since that day I was mailing a letter to them—"Dear Mommy and Daddy" and giving them lots of real love. I feel if you talk to someone else about people, you are betraying them. I probably betray myself most of all since I am always telling things about myself.

During the session though I didn't feel bad. I was much too hot—I felt like I was in leggings, a bundled up baby—and maybe I should have said something. But then I adapted myself to the heat, and the heat was a cozy pastime. I am a lazy boy fishing off a bank. If I put the right kind of mother bait on, you will always bite.

No, I know what you were trying to do. To tell me to believe in what I say. To accept the limitations and faults of my parents. But every time I do think about those things, I seem to diminish. As I take away from them, I am taking away from my-self. And also I realize I have not changed or wrestled with my parents at all.

I have told them almost everything in my life. But my life is not there, in all those facts and stories. It still feels buried. The only vital agitation I have with these facts is dreams. And then my parents and I are much more active and ghastly.

Comfort I have been trying to get is by digging down, burrow-ing back to the nest, surrounding myself with calm. I really think I must be still burrowed in the cave, like Plato's cave, since I write and think only with analogies. Everything is like something else. Even this write-up is so veiled, it is not direct. Maybe you wouldn't understand it. Here's another translation. "Yeck!" That's how my mouth and eyes and face and mind feel after I have revelled (pun—I meant to say but misspelled "revealed") just enough to keep me floundering but not drowning.

January 13

DR. YALOM

A RATHER distant hour. I felt distant from Ginny and think she probably felt distant, though not so much as I. In fact, it is only with considerable effort that I can bring myself to dictate this. There was a five-minute lag between the first and second sentence. She started off by saying she has been outside herself the past few days, and feels nervous and tense. I couldn't find any convenient way of involving her or involving myself in what was going on. I tried to get into last week, but she remembered very little from that session. She then talked about her feeling that she doesn't change. She gets to a certain point in her sexual relations with Karl but can't go any further. She's done the same in therapy with me. I tried to pry up some examples of changes that she has made, in fact, even suggested that we get out one of the old tape recordings we made a couple of years ago. She wasn't too happy about that and managed to come up with a few ways in which she felt some changes had occurred. I think I try to help Ginny find ways of discussing her progress more for my sake than for her own.

Following this she returned to her relationship with Karl. Her current plight is that she is merely marking time, waiting around to be told when it will all be over. A few days ago he gave up his business and took another job. She knows this change means something and what it may mean is that he will begin saving money to go to Mexico and then she will, one day, learn from him whether or not he intends to take her with him. If not, the relationship is over. I was rather overwhelmed with the helplessness she expressed. At the same time I realized that she takes pride in her helpless tragic pose. I even tried to bait her by referring to her as the little match girl, and then followed quickly with the suggestion that she decide, adult-like, what she wants from the relationship. Is there no decision she has to make? Is there anything in the relationship that might make *her* move to terminate it? For example, if Karl refused to support her, or if he would never permit her to have children. It was very difficult to prod her into saying that she could make a decision. In fact, it's even impossible for her to ask Karl whether he intends to take her to Mexico; she feels she has to wait in silence until he tells her. I ended up the session rather despairing and baffled about how I could infuse her with any respect for her own rights. At one point she said she tried to ask me a couple of weeks ago about my vacation and she couldn't pull it off; it would be the same thing with Karl. I suggested she try again with me. Could she now ask about my vacation or about anything else? She asked how I felt the sessions were going, but since it was already after the hour was over, we passively agreed to pick up from there next time.

January 13

GINNY

AT THE END of the session, things began when you asked me to ask you a question. It's kind of like kids miming throwing stones, and then one kid throws a real stone. At first when you said, "Ask me about the vacation," I thought I had inadvertently come up with a real piece of information that you were leaving on a big vacation. I always feel great when I am so dense and not intuitively knowing all. But that was the realest part of the session. I did ask you vis-à-vis with my eyes a few weeks ago but my talking is kind of like me alone in a rain barrel. Or a limp actress on stage talking to the audience. She can't see them because of the lights, she knows they're out there and that she must give the appearance of reaching out and making contact and looking directly in their eyes. If she needs help she must imagine them. I still haven't really spoken to you as though you are as near as you are.

And with Karl I try to be all good, simultaneously storing my mistakes in my brain. With you I try to be all bad. I say all the worst things about my situation. And neither way is realistic. I realized that last week.

I would like to flow with my moods and take from you. But instead, before I come in, I have a theme song—"I am nervous." And the overture keeps playing until in the last minute when the curtain's about to come up with your line, "Ask me a question," I notice that it's intermission for another week.

I go outside and make the air smell like popcorn for me. And I think I'm hungry and this at least is a real sensation, so I go buy a lunch with black and white soda, with expectation stretching back to when I was five years old, and a hamburger, and when I don't enjoy either, I am still paying $1.79. It strikes me like a wave—that here I am paying this money for this crap, and I have just not given you anything. (I don't mean money which I don't want to pay. I mean real feelings.)

Probably the horrible things I say in session make me feel guilty. You were right about word magic. Although when you said it, I thought you meant all the bad metaphors I used to cover up real statements.

This whole write-up for sessions is word magic which I hide. Which I wouldn't want anyone to see.

But the biggest magic that has ever entered my life is not words but real emotions and actions, like tears and thrashings. I get lost talking. I have no subtext.

I have been able to appreciate the good things that happen to me.

January 20

DR. YALOM

A RATHER important meeting. I had the feeling, it may be an illusionary one, that we broke new ground today. But then I think of the old story back at Johns Hopkins of the patients who would come in for years and almost every week the chart would say— patient better, patient better—and then at the end of several years, one sees that there really has been no change. Nevertheless, even taking this into consideration, somehow I feel that we moved into new and fertile territory today.

Things started with Ginny complaining of a very severe migraine headache. I uged her to see an internist, whereupon she quickly changed the subject and launched into a discussion she had had with a good friend, which merely reinforced some things we had talked about at our last meeting: namely, that this friend and her husband would like Ginny to visit them sometimes alone, the reason being that nobody sees much of Ginny when Karl is around. She gives herself up when he is present, becoming little more than a mute and featureless shadow. In the midst of this I tried to state very clearly, and more than once, that I thought the relationship with Karl was a limited one in which she was not herself, and, what's more, that changing might not be a way of losing the relationship but strengthening it, since I suspect that Karl, or any man, would relate more to a full woman. I also mentioned the opposite possibility; it may be that Karl has a good deal invested in her being just the way she is and any change would drive him away, in which case, I said, I'm not sure that would be particularly calamitous, since an involvement with a person who doesn't let one grow is hardly a healthy situation for either party.

She went on then to engage in some more self-derogatory sentiments. For example, she had been feeling depressed all day and rather "than staying with the feeling last night," she got dressed up very pretty and went to play pinochle at a friend's house. She called herself frivolous for that. I indicated that labelling herself as "frivolous" is another example of her semantic self-flagellation. Why not "plucky" or "resilient"?

She blocked for awhile. Then I began to prod her for her feelings toward me. She stated that she hardly ever writes about me in the post meeting write-ups, and she knows she never presents me to her friends as a real person, in fact pretends to have little allegiance to me. She added that her friends are curious about me, for example, they want to know my age. I asked her what she told them and she said "thirty-eight," and I said that was very close, that I was thirty-nine. She admitted having cleverly manipulated me into telling her my age without asking me directly. We went back to last week, when at the end of the hour I suggested she ask me something and I asked her again to do so. Then she asked how I really felt about the hours, were they O.K.? I told her that she could probably find out a lot more when she reads what I've written; basically I had mixed feelings—occasionally I felt impatient or pessimistic and often I felt good about them. She wondered how she would feel later about my saying that I was pessimistic or discouraged. I pointed out that I don't often have that feeling, and that I felt reluctant about saying that openly to her because she always presents herself as such a fragile flower, that I am afraid such a comment would leave her crushed and defenseless.

I asked her what else she wanted to ask me, and then she asked whether or not I thought of her between the sessions. I tried to rephrase that by asking if she meant whether or not I care about her. That was difficult for both of us for awhile, and she seemed on the verge of tears. Abruptly she said she doesn't really care if I care about her "in that way," but then she started to cry and confessed that she thinks about me, about parts of my body and my hair, and wondered how she's allowed me to become such an important part of her life. Also we got into a discussion of the fact that she can't really get well because if she gets well, she'll lose me, for it is unlikely that we shall continue our relationship as two equal adults. At the same time, however, she wants me to treat her like an adult, and I said to her, fearing very much that I was being a scolding parent, that to be treated like an adult, one has to act like an adult. It really came out sounding disgustingly pedantic but I didn't know quite else how to put it. I think this tact of helping her to relate to me more as a grown-up person and helping her to inquire more about my personal life is going to be useful and I'll encourage her to continue.

January 20

GINNY

OH GOD. Yesterday's session was the first that I began to feel my own methods. And why I defeat myself. I play the children's game that says "take five steps," but unless I say "may I?" I get put back or put myself back. After the session in little ways I tested my power. And that kind of extended the session further. For instance, at night when Karl wanted to read instead of going to bed, although not coming right out with it, I did tell him that there was something between reading and deep sleep.

In that one bramble bush toward the end where I said "I don't want you to like me like that but (big pause) to care for me," I started half crying. It was more like I cried because here I was back to my old cliché, "Do you like me, care for me?" I start to cry and get ashamed because I have travelled so little. Like a child who says "ma ma" up to five years old, crying in frustration because though he means "ma ma" he means a whole lot more.

When I was home I saw how my parents must have done everything for me when I was young. Comforting me even before I needed it, feeding me, buying me wonderful things. So somehow I feel like I've never made a needy gesture. Everything was just all around me in abundance. And that's the way I place myself around other people now—like a delicious fruit bowl waiting at a table, and the fruit already a little spoiled.

As with everything I seem to have gotten stuck on the sentence, "I need," or "Do you like me?" Three years ago that was revolu-

tionary for me. Just like the abundant sexual feeling and awakening I have now. But I don't extend them or draw them out any further.
What follows close behind me is my catatonic shadow that convinces me
    I do not move.
    I do not stagger on.
    I don't progress.
    I only pose, a model for my shadow,
      a shadow for my silhouette.

February 8

DR. YALOM

A RATHER unsatisfying feel for this hour. I think I've been too intrusive in forcing my values upon Ginny. I was too authoritarian today, too directive, and engaged in too much exhorting and preaching. But it was hard for me to do anything else. She began the hour by talking about her many fantasies of leaving Karl and somehow starting life anew. Over and over again, when I hear these fantasies, I can only think that there is obviously a strong part of her that wants to leave him, that is highly dissatisfied with the relationship, or that perceives the relationship as a stifling one. Then she described an incident in which Karl suggested to her that she share the gasoline money with him. He is now earning approximately $90 a week, she only $30. She does the cooking, grocery shopping, and the cleaning, and though she feels it's unfair for her to have to pay gasoline money as well, she made only a feeble protest to his request and ended up by consenting.

I tried to make her see that giving in to something she considers unfair stems from a refusal to recognize her own rights. I feel that in the long run this is self-destructive; she's almost insuring that Karl, if he's a well-integrated person, will soon tire of their relationship. If, on the other hand, he's the kind of person who really needs such a selfless, disenfranchised friend, then he's going to stay permanently. But either way it's self-destructive. She said that she would not like to continue this relationship permanently, but that it's very sweet in some ways. Without him, life would be an abyss; without him, she'd fall apart. I told her I thought that was bullshit and she agreed, although the abysmal feeling is very real. I then asked her what she would have to do to change things and she went over, in a rather effective fashion, the types of things she would say to him and his response, which would generally end up with his lowering the boom on her and concluding that they should break up.

Unfortunately, however, the treatment hour took on the aura of a pep talk, in which I was urging her to do things she may not be ready to do; yet somehow I want to impart to her the knowledge and the feeling that is really *her* responsibility to change her life. It may be that Karl is such a limited person that they will break up, and I guess I feel in the long run that's just as well. On the other hand, I could imagine that Karl or any man would be really impressed at her gradually growing up and becoming a "mensch" and if that's too much for him to handle, so be it. I'm sure Ginny in the long run will find plenty of other men who can appreciate her as a more integrated person.

February 8

GINNY

IT'S HARD for me to remember what happened. It all seemed pretty direct and straightforward (a cliché, that sentence like "How are you?"). When I go in to the session like that—full of grievances that have been aching all day—I feel like I have a deficiency, like a vitamin one, and you have to supply the stuff that gets my complaints out, that stops the cracked record from repeating.

I think you probably got to see more of me as others see me, or as I function, in that session. I don't really try to interact

with people, I intuit or imagine what their behavior and circumstances will be, and improvise my responses out of nervous
energy. No thought process anywhere. Like for instance when
I was sure that you would only have the 1-2 hour slot free, and
built a labyrinth of arguments around it. I kind of evolve all
convoluted.

It was the first time in therapy you didn't side with me—you
know how you said, "Well any man would leave a woman who
only showed the surface." I liked that.

I think Karl really is a good strong person. And he is only
stingy because he is not in love. If he did love me, things would
come naturally—the gasoline would flow without me having to
make a federal case out of it. I guess I am really hurt because
in putting down petty rules for Karl and me, I know I am asking
them to take the place of love and generosity.

When I finally told Karl, it was anti-dramatic. He said he didn't
like the martyr quality in me. "Behind every martyr is a shrew."
He says he only wants to be told things and that's true. When I
tell him something immediately, he's very pliable, acquiesces,
doesn't put up a fight, provided my voice comes out deep and
resonant. However, as soon as I delay the emotion, and then
replay it, if he detects the slightest screechy timbre to my voice,
he turns on me, and whatever point I've won, I've also lost.

And the dialogue never got as deep as I had planned. But it
was still better to get it out.

February 17

DR. YALOM

I HAD a patient immediately after Ginny and some unusual scheduling difficulties which didn't permit me to dictate a note on her. Now
it's been several days and the interview has begun to blur in my mind.
The most striking thing was that she came in and immediately
said, "Well, don't you want to hear what happened?" and then went
on to tell me that she had talked to Karl about the things we had

discussed last time. It hadn't worked out too well, because Karl got a little upset with her acting like a martyr all the time, but, in fact, I think in many ways it did work out, because she doesn't have to pay for the gasoline and has been able to assert herself, if only minimally. I was a bit surprised that she came in that strong because I hadn't really sensed she was going to go ahead and literally do some of the things we had discussed last time.

At some point in the interview I wondered what she wanted to work on next. She talked about making love and wanting to be able to ask for things for herself. I wondered what she wanted to be able to ask for. What Ginny said then was so benign that she couldn't help laughing at herself: she merely wanted to ask Karl to do something a little longer because it felt good. I asked her to say this aloud a couple of times, so that she could take some distance from it and see the absurdity of her inability to say this, and she could not repeat her statement without mimicking herself or saying it with a funny accent.

She also expressed the feeling that what she has with Karl is very precious and I am going to take it away from her somehow. When she was lying in his arms in the morning, she realized how much this means to her and that nothing else is really as important. Ginny also felt rather proud of herself because she had had a migraine the night before, hadn't taken any strong drug for it, and somehow managed to triumph over the headache without being all drugged up today.

It's remarkable how four days later I can't go back and really recapture what my feelings were to her during the hour. They all blur into a generalized good feeling, and I know that she was happy and bouncy during the session. Of course, I always like to see her like that. Now I do remember that we talked about how young she felt. She does manifest herself to me often like a very young girl. I also remember that, as usual, she shouldered all the blame for therapy sessions which she considers unsatisfactory. Obviously there must be times when she is dissatisfied with what I give her, and she rather tenuously got into the area by admitting she sometimes wishes I could show her more of myself. I asked her what kinds of things she wanted to know, but we didn't get very far with that question.

February 17

GINNY

WHEN I came yesterday I was expecting a surprise. Something that would make the session a little different. An emotional assignment. The expectation of going cured a migraine. My fantasy and release kept step with my walking as I rounded the long path to the hospital. I am always "cured" and jubilant on the walk in, and feel about as heavy as a piece of duck down.

I say things in therapy that are not true. Even as I'm saying them, I know I don't believe them, that they will confuse you. Like when I said, "you're sitting across from me and seeing nothing." Many times you've told me you don't think of me as nothing. If only I could catch myself when I'm saying things like that, contradict myself, say "No that's not what I mean," maybe then I could take myself seriously when I speak. I don't fight for my words. They just come. That's why I tend to disbelieve them. And you diminish in my eyes when I see you going after my words too seriously—some of my words.

You said one thing yesterday that I had never thought of before and therefore came as a revelation—that if I am so scared to say "such benign things, they must be substitutes for angrier things hiding." I don't know if they are angrier things or just stronger things. Like not saying "I love you" to K, when I sometimes feel it.

Anyway all the energy I have, even yesterday, seems to be wasted on observation. And yet it's not observation of a present moment, but big memory observation, years of experience that I can tally with one sarcasm. And when good things come up they hardly penetrate my way of looking. I am what I see, not what others see in me, but what I see. I feel very removed. Maybe that's why I can't get close to you with words. Cause I can't get close enough to myself with words. If these write-ups were intellectual, that'd be one thing. But I don't even think in them.

They're automatic. They're like not carrying a problem into therapy and waiting for your surprise agenda to save the day. Lately you've been putting slight pressure on me to do things. Like thinking about the gasoline. I appreciate this. Because every small thing I do gives me more to work with, more exposure, and disappointment, cause it is still one removed, not originating with me. Coming from you.

February 24

DR. YALOM

THE MEETING started off in black despair. Ginny said she had been up almost all night, because of a terribly upsetting incident which centered around Karl's saying to her that she was, in effect, "a sexual lump." I remember Nietzsche's statement that the very first time you meet someone you know all about him, and from that point on you gradually erase these correct impressions. My first response to her description of the incident was that it corroborated my first impressions of Karl; it was a horridly callous remark and should have called forth some anger in Ginny. She went on describing it in some detail, I got sucked up into her pathos, and considered with her ways to break through the impasse that had developed between them. It seems that she had, earlier in the evening, perhaps unwittingly rejected his advances, and thus felt responsible for his reaction and, in fact, totally accepted his definition of her as a lump. She began feeling like a lump in all aspects of her being despite the fact that Ginny is anything but a lump. She is alive, imaginative, deeply creative, and very bouncy. Indeed, earlier that day she had gotten dressed in some outlandish spoof costume just to amuse Karl and later had gotten into a long giggling spree in a German class they had attended together. All this stands out in marked contrast to seeing herself as a lump.

All I could do at this point was to question her willingness to accept another person's definition of her. She lives in constant terror

55

that suddenly Karl will announce the news that he is through with her. She was so afraid that Karl was thinking about the relationship last night, because, if he thought about it, then that would be curtains for her; so she partially felt that she wanted to interrupt his thought processes. Once again no recognition that she has any rights or any choice in the relationship.

Gradually, however, I returned to my feelings about her anger. In her fantasies during that night she once again imagined leaving Karl and even committing suicide. In a dream she and Karl were being pursued, and Karl was killed. I commented that, although she claims to feel no anger toward Karl, she killed him off in the dream. She pointed out that they were together and that she begged for his life to be spared, but I think that was irrelevant. The important thing is that she expresses some of her anger in her fantasies and dreams, but is absolutely unable to do so consciously. As we talked, she remembered a fleeting feeling, a whispered hope that Karl might apologize to her in the morning, and I tried to make her recognize that hidden part of herself which felt offended and expected an apology. But there was no way in which I could help her overtly experience any of her anger toward Karl, even in play acting. As a rehearsal exercise, I suggested she try to express some of her disappointment with me. This was quite hard for her to do. We ended the hour with her feeling that she had failed once again. I tried to reassure her with the explanation that we had gotten into a really crucial area for her—one which we'll have to work on for a long period of time: her inability to express any anger, or aggression, and her inability to assert herself and demand her rights all fit together in this gestalt. What stops her from feeling anger, let alone expressing it, is something we haven't even begun to explore. I've got a hunch she has a brimming, but hidden reservoir of anger, but is fearful of tapping it lest she be unable to turn off the spigot. At one point I even taunted her with the question, "Could it be that sweet little Ginny wants to murder somebody?" But I got no response.

February 24

GINNY

DURING the session, a part of me was really getting excited, but it was surrounded by the therapy character who sits on the leather chair and listens and thinks "maybe." And on cue concludes tamely that nothing really happened, though there is still a possibility.

When you kept wanting me to go after anger and I couldn't, I felt miserable inside but I also felt "very adult" sitting there on the outside. It was almost like you were interviewing the parent and the child.

I would listen to the little thing inside and then I would tell you about it once removed. Inside I was boundless, saying things like—"Fuck you. Fuck him. Fuck him." But it would just sit there. Never really talking itself because if it would, it couldn't use the same kinds of words I do or the dubbed conversational tone.

I pose as heavier and "stronger" and "more conventional" than the small anger or sadness inside. Which would dribble out, wet my eyes, be mostly incoherent, attack the things that go round in my memory. It's like when you say, "Maybe Ginny's so angry she wants to kill." I agree with you—we're like two women at a park and one has the child on a leash and there are so many things—swings, jungle jims—the child could get into, and we discuss abstractly those things. I feel a slight tugging on the leash, like a man who goes fishing to sleep on the shore with the sun and some beer. He feels a pull, smiles, dozes and lets the fish nibble and go. I always feel the little pull in our sessions.

Sometimes, like that night before, I feel desperate and tired. But I never really catch what has been biting and gnawing at the line. I just get calm again and it is gone, the terrifying feelings, the helplessness.

You gave me a great deal of hope and confidence when you said that you had started to see me and my problems more clearly and that we were just at the beginning and would have a lot more chances. That is the leather chair persona thanking you while the squirt inside me is still ranting: Fuck you. Fuck him.

March 3

DR. YALOM

A WORKDAY, bread and butter session. Ginny started by telling me that she had been thinking about the content of our last meeting, especially about her inability to express anger, which she recognizes as very true indeed. Not only is she unable to voice her anger, but she is terribly uncomfortable around other people who can and do. She then described a conversation with Karl following our last session, in which he, as he often does, asked her what we talked about, and wondered whether it had been about the previous night. This surprised me somewhat because it seems as though Karl is much more closely attuned to their relationship than she sometimes implies. He was giving her a perfect opportunity to talk about her anguish, which she did to some extent, saying that she didn't like being called a lump, but he pointed out that when he said this, she didn't do anything—just lay there and became even more like a lump. This, to me, tended to confirm what I've been suggesting to Ginny for some time—that her fear of expressing anger because it might endanger her relationship with Karl (or someone else) does in fact bring about the very thing she dreads, i.e., a stunted or severely damaged human relationship. By not giving vent to her anger and other profound emotions, by remaining a one-dimensional person, she prevents people from relating to her with the kind of depth and egalitarianism she would prefer. If Karl leaves her, it will not be because she has driven him away with her anger, but with her lack of anger. I wondered whether she has always been like that. Ginny said "yes" and gave a couple of examples when she did express some anger but shook with terror during the act. She pointed out that during her childhood her mother usually expressed her anger for her.

I said that perhaps one of the things she could do would be to start talking about her feelings toward me, which might be easier than with Karl. She nodded, as though that were very logical, but when I asked her to talk about some of the things that she disliked most in me, it was extraordinarily difficult for her to say anything, although we've been through this several times already. The criticisms she selected were thinly veiled virtues. For example, one of my problems is patience; I am too patient with her. Most of the things she said were based on the premise of my omniscience. She stated that I really knew everything that was going on but there were times in the therapy group when she wished I had acted in such a way as to satisfy the needs of certain members, even though that may not have been what they needed in the long run. I pointed out that she attributed more omniscience to me than I possessed and that there were times, in fact, when I really didn't know what the hell was going on with some of the group members or with Ginny, for that matter. She reacted as though that were really news to her.

Next she mentioned a couple of other things; she wished that I could reveal more of my feelings, that I could show more annoyance with her, but she's not sure whether I wouldn't just be like her mother at that point. She talked again about how upset she feels when Karl is not sleeping because she thinks he is contemplating leaving her. I felt frustrated, caught again in a vicious circle, and could only comment that her worrying about Karl's leaving her causes her to be tense and anxious, which in turn will promote the very thing she fears. I wondered whether the same pattern occurred in her conversations with me: that she was so worried about my leaving her that she has to be careful about what she says. She denied that, but later asked, in a whisper, what was going to happen to our sessions after the summer. I pretended that I didn't hear her so as to make her phrase the question a little more clearly; in other words what I wanted her to do was get some experience in asking a straightforward question, which is entirely her right to ask. So what she did was to ask me, "Will you continue seeing me after June?" I answered that I would. I asked whether there was anything else she wanted to ask me and she said "no." She talked about the lack of personal feeling she's had toward me, unlike her strong interest in other people in her life, such as some of her teachers. When she discusses her therapy with one of her friends, she usually describes me in impersonal terms.

Somehow we began to speak again of her sexual feelings toward Karl and her inability to initiate any sexual activity, although Karl had recently "given her permission" to make sexual demands on him. She talked about her sexual tensions during the day and her ability to deal with them rather quickly by masturbation, since I had assured her it was okay. It seems as though my attempts to take some of her guilt and anxiety out of the masturbatory act were successful.

I had planned to see her next week, even though I couldn't make it on our normal Wednesday, but as she wasn't necessarily expecting it and had made some other plans, I finally decided that, since next week is so hectic, we'll skip the session.

March 3

GINNY

OF COURSE I have waited too long to write this. (It's Monday morning, nearly a week gone by.) I remember we talked about honesty, anger, speaking up.

The next night Karl was restless which was a contagious condition. I couldn't calm him or sleep myself. The anxiety and sense that I should be doing something was too much to allow for sleep.

So while I hear things in therapy, and am kind of buoyed up by the hope it gives me, when the time comes for applying them, I stay with my old patterns. They are already there, in remote control.

When you asked me to tell you my bad feelings and opinions of you, I sort of did it more intellectually than emotionally.

I know all the ways to describe my fiascoes. Describing anything else would be a new experience.

While I appear to go about with a selfless face, I am really more selfish than Karl. I don't even think that what I am doing can have some effect on him, good or bad. And so I hold back energy and keep us both as static as myself. I do it with you too, lots of times. I give you nothing but run-down sentences to work with. And then lead you on by saying I am going to try harder next time, to take it more seriously. So while I asked you if you would continue therapy with me, I sort of knew you would, and that if you didn't, only I could be hurt and I would know how to take that hurt and make it something I could bear (bare). And this kind of maneuvering of experiences, so they all get absorbed by my great fiasco digestive tract, leaves me babbling along to people who are never as real as they really are, and my self is only half realized and not going forward.

I will try to do better in the therapy reports. I think the reason they are so hard is that I'm not on multi-levels (fear is the great leveler) so that when I comment on things in the reports, I think they must be obvious or already said.

March 17

DR. YALOM

WE DID NOT meet last week. Ginny started off the session by saying that she had spent last Wednesday (our usual meeting day) with friends. Her friend, who had just finished a long workshop for changing her own behavior, spent about five hours working on Ginny. Ginny felt she was being strangled by this girl. I felt that she was implying that she had already been strangled by me. We returned to familiar ground, i.e., Ginny's inability to express anger. It's becoming clearer and clearer, I think, to Ginny and to me that this seems to be a major conflict area. It's also becoming clear that whenever she gets close to expressing any anger she bursts into tears. She's done this on several occasions during the week. I told her that I thought her behavior was perfectly explicable if we accepted the assumption that she is harboring a murderous degree of rage and has to be terribly careful not to let any of it leak out. This didn't seem to mean much to her but she started to talk a bit about "petty grudges, petty rages, bits and pieces of anger" that she had toward people. She expresses them very reluctantly and in a pathetically ineffective manner. For example, she got angry at the girl who spent five hours working on her and Ginny punished her by withholding the news that she had gotten a post card from a mutual friend. Ordinarily she would have told the girl right away but this time conveyed the message twenty-four hours later. Then she confessed a sense of hopelessness and wondered if she can ever change. I questioned her definition of "change." She sees change as looming so large and issuing such radical proclamations that she must become an entirely different kind of person, and this, of course, scares her.

At this point she said she feels guilty about the lousy write-ups she's been handing in to me. I told her if she really wants to stop feeling guilty, she should write better reports. She knows this, of course, but really wants to hear me punish her for it. I wondered about the subterranean world she says she writes in; what does she hear? What happens there? What does she not say in my office? She went on talking about her sexual feelings, that she felt somewhat sexually stimulated coming in here now and it was a kind of a different feeling than usual, an adult sexual feeling. Somehow it involved me but she couldn't quite bring herself to say so, nor could she admit having any sexual fantasies about me, since that embarrasses her so much. I imagine it is awfully unfair for me to expect her to talk about her sexual fantasies toward me when I would not be willing to talk about my sexual fantasies toward her. In fact, I don't have any overt sexual fantasies about her, but I can easily push myself into feeling quite pleasant about touching Ginny or holding Ginny, although I guess the professional role is so deeply ingrained in me that I have difficulty extending the fantasy to sexual intercourse with her. However, I think that part of the shame she feels results from the inequality of a relationship, where I'm expecting her to talk about fantasies, yet not sharing in them; so in a sense the shame is to be expected and I was being unfair in urging her to talk about them. Ginny keeps insinuating that somehow or other I should be pressing her harder, that I should do something more dramatic. Sometimes I get the notion that a really good therapist would, at this point, tell Ginny she has three months to make some change or end therapy; I wonder whether it's because I like Ginny so much and enjoy working with her that I refuse to use our relationship as a fulcrum for demanding change. Am I impeding her progress by not being harsh or "therapeutic"?

March 17

GINNY

I HAVE an impression that I talked a lot. I came in with a wild nervous energy. In my dreams I had been a loved woman having affairs, and this made me happy, satisfied and aggressive as soon as I got up. When you were five minutes late for the session, I started to get angry, because I wanted to see you, didn't want to be sent home. And I fantasized that you had left for lunch partially forgetting me, and later leaving word for me to come back tomorrow. And I said (knowing I shouldn't be angry since you were doing me the favor and not vice versa) to forget it, that I would just come the next week. See I'm getting emotions but they're all evolving from fantasies or turning into fantasies.

Anyway I'm glad I at least talked in your office. A lot of times you say "I don't follow you," and usually those times are when I'm not making real sense—bull shitting, and reminiscing, using my fantasies as the experience. Like when I said I felt like a forty-five year old woman, and that everything was over for me.

When I told you about Eve's coaching me on bringing out more of my feelings and self in conversation rather than just relying on impressions and punch lines, I didn't equal the feelings that I had had that day. (You see I thought that the closed trap I was in was just with you, that with you and sometimes Karl I withheld things. But then I found I was doing it with my best friend too and being put down for. it.) I couldn't recapture for you the anxiety it gave me. But maybe that is my mistake in therapy —to think that I must produce everything I've experienced or feel I should have experienced. To keep going over experiences verbatim with no relief. Most times I think I'm not giving you the real thing and not giving it to myself. I have this precious museum of emotions and I relegate all my feelings to the few sparse exhibits, rather than letting them flow or change. That first time I ever spoke to you, three years ago, was the perfect time. (I was ripe from intense therapy and awakening.) All my emotions since then seem to be dwindling away from that vibrant moment, when I felt I spoke to you in truth and vulnerability. After being mirrored * in group therapy for two years, I'm always self-conscious in there with you now. I have an image of me, rather *than just experiencing myself*. I feel generally stagnant, all damned up. Whenever I say something it is usually very premeditated or fluff. Either way I feel I am not digging down into any new sources. I don't surprise myself most times and I'm sure I don't surprise you. This makes me angry at you, but angrier at me. I'm the one who has blocked up the current, only allowing a small seepage of feeling to escape. And when it does, I stare at it till it dries up or you do. I don't know what has made me so self-conscious. Maybe part of it is seeing myself through Karl's strong severe eyes.

I'm released from this self-consciousness—when I'm having fun with Karl or friends or you ask a question that is right. When I become involved and am not worrying about every response and what I must do. Then I miss a lot, but I feel more and usually have less memory. I get off clean. The moment and experiences seem finally over, without any bad echoes.

In therapy I can't marvel at your reactions to my controlled givings. I don't give you a live person to work with. At least this is the way I perceive it today. Even when I feel other things, this other critical image of myself is superimposed and locked in place. When I'm as nervous as I was today, it's like a television picture jumping up and down. It's the same old soap opera but it wouldn't stand still.

Maybe that fantasy about making love *and talking* at the same time is a fantasy about therapy too. That you would talk me into giving way, freeing my feelings, giving liberty to other feelings besides defeat. Usually when you say, "What do you feel for

---

* Literally, before a glass curtain with an audience of doctors.

me?" I go through this quick hard thought process—Oh there he is again trying to get me to admit I have sexual feelings toward him. Well I don't (quick answer). But today when you said it, I thought about it and allowed myself to fantasize and I did have such feelings. Though they were a free flow exercise and not something that is strongly lodged in my mind.

I seem to be more on my guard in therapy than anywhere else. Even though I know it would make you happy for me to act a little different. I don't.

Part of the defeat I feel is being able to deceive you and not get booed. I acted on the stage and somehow my face and body are superficially there whenever I want them. They put in an appearance, they understudy for emotion and strength. This gives me no good feelings though. However after therapy I am usually more able to act out my aggressions which are a retaliation against my posing.

April 14

DR. YALOM

I HAVE NOT seen Ginny for three weeks. The last two weeks I have been in Boston. The week before that I was supposed to meet Ginny at 11:00 and catch a 2:00 o'clock plane to the East Coast. I planned to do this until Tuesday when I really began to see that it was impossible for me to get everything done in time to catch that last flight out for Boston. I worked all day Tuesday and late into Tuesday evening and finally after a great deal of hesitation I decided that I had to call Ginny up Tuesday night and cancel the appointment. I still gave her the option on the phone of letting her know that if it were an absolute emergency, I would still try to swing some time to see her. Her response at that point on the phone was that it was too bad she wasn't going to meet with me because she had a good report to give me. I felt badly at missing this, frankly because I was curious to see what had happened, but at any rate that's the background for this meeting today, which I can aptly entitle "The Two-Day High."

Essentially what Ginny told me was that for a couple of days she had felt extremely well—that it seemed to have begun perhaps on Sunday evening with Karl again calling her a lump, accusing her of going right to sleep every night and not really caring for him, and she apparently retorted directly, returning anger for anger. The following morning she was able to be angry at a schoolboy who had been disobedient and taunted her on her job. No matter that she scolded the wrong boy, she was still able to find the right one and scold him, and no matter that he still didn't pay any attention to her. She began to feel very strong and potent and take herself very seriously. It sounds as if Ginny had a glimpse of her inner strength and form, and then suddenly my cancelling the interview took everything away from her. She said that she had a feeling that somehow she was going to be able to come in and get some renewal from me that would keep the current going and that my going away in a sense put an end to the circuit. She couldn't fully express these things to me on the phone because when I called she was just a couple of feet away from Karl with whom she was playing liar dice. This placed her in a rather difficult position between the two men in her life, and she whispered into the phone that she couldn't really share these recent changes with Karl because they wouldn't make any sense for him.

All of this was said in a rather brilliant fashion. Ginny was quite perky and even though she talked about this good feeling as belonging to the past, it seemed to me as if it were at least partially still present. I had a lot of thoughts about what she said and tried to explore them all systematically.

First, I wondered about the annoyance she must have felt toward me for cancelling our session. She couldn't get too far with that, of course, and I almost had to say some things for her, such as: one would have thought that I could have planned my day a little better, or that if I really cared for her, I would have tried to see her. She had thought of some of these things but then let me off with the excuse that I had to cancel everyone. At first she thought it was because she wasn't paying me, but then dismissed that interpretation by saying that I was cancelling all my paying patients too. This incidently indicates to me that I keep overlooking the whole question of Ginny's not being charged, which is much less important to me because the money my other patients pay does not go directly to me anyway but to the University, and perhaps I am not making this clear enough to Ginny, placing her more in my debt than is really the case.

Another thing I tried to investigate was the meaning of the fact that her good feelings vanished with my inability to see her. I told her that I had the fantasy of a young child performing fancy dives on the diving board and saying all the while to his mother "watch me, watch me," and when suddenly after a half hour he realizes that his mother hasn't really been watching him, this strips the pleasure from the entire procedure. In other words, it is lamentable that Ginny has to feel good only for me. She denied this, insisting she felt good for herself as well, but something was missing; my interpretation was that she felt I didn't care enough.

A lot of other things are going on in her life now that are upsetting her. She must move from the house in which she is living, since her landlord and his wife have just gotten a divorce and everything, including the furniture she has been using for the past year, is being sold very quickly; Ginny immediately berates herself for not dealing with this in a superhuman fashion. She has volunteered to help the landlord who is incapacitated with sickness, and then criticizes herself for not fulfilling this function with total equanimity, when of course anyone would be upset for having to give up things he had lived with and loved, including the landlord. It is characteristic of Ginny to take almost any happening as a sign of her own inferiority or lack of grace. She feeds the events of her day into a self-critical mill churned by the power of her own self-hatred. I talked about this, pointing out some of the "shoulds" which govern her self-perception and impose superhuman demands. She spoke about a girlfriend's visit and I tried to make her see their meeting from the viewpoint of her friend; Ginny is aware of the fact that the girlfriend thinks highly of her. I know that Ginny must be constantly exposed to a great many good feelings about herself—the good feelings that I have about her are shared, I suspect, by most of the people who have continued contact with her, and I wondered with her why all of these good feelings from others somehow never make a dent on her basic core of self-hatred. That's about where we ended the session today.

Perhaps a bit more than before, I begin to see some light at the end of the labyrinth. The mere fact that Ginny was able to have a two-day high is very heartening. Sometimes a patient can hold inside himself this kind of experience as a reference point for future progress, recognizing familiar terrain when he gets near again. Ginny now tends to do the very opposite. She remembers this peak and immediately realizes how dead she is the rest of the time. However, I think we'll be back at this point again many times in the future.

———

April 21

D.R. YALOM

GINNY came in extremely distraught today. Furthermore, I was between 10 and 15 minutes late, which obviously didn't help matters. I felt somewhat guilty during the meeting for having been late because this was not the day to have been late for Ginny. On the other hand, maybe it wasn't harmful since it helped her mobilize her anger a bit toward me. I was harried by the architects in planning the new psychiatric building across the street, and as I was leaving today for a few days, they kept pushing me over the time limit, but still my lateness was not absolutely unavoidable. At any rate Ginny really feels as though she's slipped back several notches. She feels at her very worst. What happened is that she's been under a tremendous amount of pressure. She must find a new apartment to live in within a week, all of her furniture is being sold out from under her, Karl severly burned his hand because of her negligence in the kitchen, she hasn't been able to write for three weeks, etc. etc. I felt concerned about her increased distress this week and told her so. I'm sure that when the dust settles, she'll feel a lot more comfortable. However, I think it's quite important now to see clearly what she does to herself during times of stress.

What she does is to start doing things for everyone else, then she wallows in a great deal of self-pity, and perhaps makes herself so pitiable that she ends up being rejected by others. What's different this time, however, is the nature of her rage, which is much closer to the surface. Usually she swallows it deeply and then feels bewildered and helpless with her never expressed, never acted upon anger. She talked about how angry she was at having to come down to see me today. Though I was trying to pull her out of the mud, nevertheless she had too much to do to take this much time out of her life and get sick on the bus to boot. Furthermore, she woke up with thoughts of owning a gun and shooting people. When she went to ask the secretary where I was, she had the feeling that if I missed today's session, it would be a fitting caption for the week. She had a little trouble opening the glass window at the office and a strong impulse to ram her fist through the glass. Karl had been thoughtless, pushing her to go look at apartments when she was too tired to move and making her go to a bookstore when she didn't want to, then scolding her for not having dinner ready, though in jest. Shortly after that she accidentally left a red-hot pan on the counter and he burned himself; for a moment she had thought it was poetic justice, and hated herself for that. (Obviously it is less "poetic justice" than destructive impulses breaking repressive barriers). She had been aware that it was unwise to leave this pan on the counter, thought it was dangerous to leave matches next to it, but somehow managed to push it out of her mind within a couple of minutes. She was angry with her father today, and even with me, although she wasn't able to talk about this too freely.

There was so much going on, I had difficulty knowing what I could do to help her; and at the end of the session I had the distinct feeling that I hadn't been very useful. Ginny walked out looking somewhat discouraged and downcast, probably with the feeling that it had been a long trip to see me for no real profit.

During the interview I had tried to make her realize that the situation was not out of control as she imagined it to be: she retained her freedom of choice in each instance and could take any of these problems one by one and think of corrective moves. With some minor effort, for example, she could correct her own untidiness and the messy rooms. However, she seemed much too distraught for such practical suggestions to have any effect. Furthermore, she stated that she was too harried this week to write up anything for me—she had said everything she wanted to say last week and if she had anything more to say, she would say it to my face. This sounded awfully challenging to me, and I tried to help her move more deeply into the feeling but she wouldn't. I think that she may well be nourishing some anger toward me for having missed several weeks ago. She said she knew I would say this, but that it wasn't true; in fact, it was silly to look back to the events of a month ago when there were so many urgent things going on in her life.

At any rate, I had some contact with the old Ginny today, a return to discouragement, pessimism, and puzzlement on my part and to Ginny's feelings of shame about her messiness and sloppiness; we were both sucked into her pit of self-abasement.

May 5

DR. YALOM

GINNY started off by saying she didn't have her report, she didn't have time to do it, but then muttered under her breath that she did have time to go to the races. When I questioned her, she insisted she really was much too busy, every moment of her time had been spent in packing and moving, and any free time she gave herself was a necessary respite from the household situation. She was depressed, not much was happening, she had said everything there was to be said at the last meeting. All of this left me disgruntled and I felt an urge to scold her for not writing the report, since that's her part of the contract she made with me. In fact, I even considered telling her that if she wasn't going to keep up her end of the contract, I wouldn't keep up mine. But that would make the writing extremely coercive and mechanical, and I also hesitated from saying this because she was so dreadfully down. For the next twenty or twenty-five minutes, we had an extremely dull session. It was mainly a rehash of things she's talked about before. I don't think she uttered one fresh or refreshing phrase. Mainly she served up once again a nondescript selection of drab morsels from her self-negating smorgasbord.

I tried to find a way to cut into this constructively, but I was simply unable to say anything to her during the first part of the interview. There was nothing I could think of that would be very useful, nothing that I particularly felt like exploring or reinforcing; so I found myself, quite against my will, rather silent. I pointed out to her that she was being very little-girlish, that she was speaking in a feeble timid manner and saying nothing new. She responded by agreeing. She then told me a fantasy that she had had in the morning. The fantasy had to do with my sending her to a little cottage instructing her to write, and then my helper came along and had sexual relations with her, which provided quite a jolly romp. After awhile, however, sex with the helper got to be more than just fun in that it turned into incessant intercourse on the verge of rape. She was then tempted to run away with him; however, I came and persuaded her to stay with the writing for at least another month or so. We explored the fantasy—did she really want me to take care of her in a neat little cottage and even provide for her sexual needs? It was a real mothering task that she was asking of me. What are some of the things she would want me to ask about? (I always find it illuminating to ask patients what questions they would like me to ask them.) She found herself unable to answer except to suggest I tell her more things to do or ask her more specific questions about her shift in moods. She also wanted me to tell her what to do.

I then proceeded for the last fifteen minutes of the interview to be a Mother-extreme. For example, she had said that one thing she liked was when I suggested she go on the train and she had gone on the train last time. I asked her whether she went on the train today— she said no, and I asked her why not, and we went into the details of why she hadn't caught the train today. Then I asked her exactly what she had done today, and she told me what time she woke up and what she was thinking about. I asked her what she did then and she talked about her washing and the fact that she hadn't washed very well and I pursued this by asking if she would like me to wash her and she said no, but she'd like me to give her a "free shower." It was a funny choice of words, the "free" made no sense; however, I couldn't find out any more about that. She then talked about break-fast, saying that she really wanted cereal and strawberries, but wouldn't permit herself to have that, even though it may have meant that the strawberries would remain uneaten and become rotten. She says it's just one of the ways she has of depriving herself of what she wants. Her mother in the past would help her decide what kind of food to eat. I persisted in this line of questioning for awhile and we ended the interview with my suggesting to her that she *should* have the strawberries and cereal tomorrow, and that she *should* take the train next time.

This certainly livened things up in the interview. At one point she said she felt very hot, almost like a sexual hotness, and then went on from there to talk about something that sounded quite curious and rather intriguing; she had almost decided today that she was not going to let me get to her and that she was going to remain in control of me by being untouchable. She remembered being that way in the group—aloof and emotionally unreachable. I asked her more about how that would make me feel toward her. She said that the only word that came to mind was "in awe of." This seems to suggest that by not being touched, by remaining somewhat dead, she manages to control me and perhaps, through her frigidity, Karl. There is a tight, defiant fist inside that fuzzy mitten.

May 18

DR. YALOM

THIS WAS a very tense, unsettling interview. First of all, today was the day we exchanged our written reports of the last few months. I haven't done too much thinking about them except to tell the secretary to get the write-ups together. This morning I was going to spend some time reading mine and perhaps editing them to make them more intelligible to Ginny, since I haven't been proofing them after dictation. As I started reading, I became more and more embarrassed and asked myself what on earth I was doing showing all of these to Ginny and wondered what their effect would be on her. I finally resolved all of this by stopping after reading a couple of the write-ups. I also glanced over a couple of Ginny's in the process but didn't read hers systematically either, since I felt we both ought to do that together this week and talk about it next time. One thing that was evident to me was that in one sense the tables are turned—Ginny often sees me as having the upper hand and yet when we look at the use of language, it is quite clear that my language is clumsy and unimaginative as compared to hers. At the beginning of the interview I felt more and more apprehensive about the wisdom of sharing these with Ginny, and told her that if she were so upset by the reports that she had to call me, I would be available. She also seemed uneasy about reading them and, amusingly enough, considered putting a comic book cover around them so that Karl wouldn't know what she was reading.

Ginny came in looking very well today. She had called and switched days so she could come a day earlier because Karl was going to be driving her down today. The whole meeting was rather tense and a lot of the tension was of a sexual nature. Ginny talked about her intense sexual feelings, which seemed to circulate around me or at least be tangential to me. When I asked her whether feeling sexy was in any way related to seeing me today, she would go from there to talk of masturbation, with a sense of gratitude for my having given her permission, almost as if I were a priest-pardoner.

Then she talked about how upset she felt at calling me yesterday to change the hour, how it was like her mother who had once forced her to call boys on Sadie Hawkins day. I commented on the fact that in the last session she had talked about having sex with my delegate or helper. She said that if she could tell Karl everything she has been able to tell me, she'd feel much more easy and would probably be able to allow herself greater sexual freedom with him. I wondered if an extension of this line of thought might be that if she were to have sexual relations with me, she would be able to unblock herself further yet. She said she sometimes thinks of that but doesn't really permit herself to think about it for long or to fantasize it. I suggested that she does at a subintellectual level, since she gets flooded with sexual tension when she comes into the office. I wondered if talking about it would help to exorcise the tension which was present and which did seem to be blocking her today.

We had a hard time getting through the hour. Time seemed to drag. Maybe it was the expectation of reading the reports. We discussed the way she looked in her mini-dress, which she considered much too short; she felt embarrassed about it, sorry she had worn it or sorry she had not worn long pants with it. I asked what she thought my reaction to her dress was. She didn't take me up on this and I gratuitously told her that I hadn't noted any of the unflattering things she was saying, that it looked fine to me. I wondered too if her high sexual tension today had something to do with Karl and me, both being in Palo Alto today; she seems to feel very much caught between us. I didn't say this, though; I'm sure it would have been of little use.

I'm quite curious about her summaries and her response to mine. Next week seems a long time away.

May 18

GINNY

I SHOULD have written my report before I started reading your reports. But anyway I had a fantasy in the session last time—it belongs to my vulgar dreams. See I was so nervous and thought that if I could have masturbated before or right there, I would be relieved and could get on to the business at hand. This bizarre thought had overtones and in fact was plagiarized from a scene in *The Story of O* where a girl does it in her office on a swivel chair in front of a man. But this really wasn't what I was feeling. I'm not sure if all of the above is real or just a clever pastime to get out of concentrating. When I go blank, I try to align my thoughts to things I've read in books—secondary sources of experience.

However, what was real is that when I do personal things, I imagine you there lots of times. So in my transparency I couldn't see what would be the difference if you were there in my mind or were really there. At home, for instance, you sometimes appear. I talk to you. That day in session it was like coming in with a stomach-ache. It was just a practical remedy, I thought. I had all that nervous energy and no sanctuary. And your office is like a sanctuary for me—where I can say some of the things I need to, with amnesty, without fear of being judged. When I need privacy other times, I station you by my bedroom door, or next to my bed. Kind of like a psychological bouncer. You watch over me, protecting and listening. Or if I run away, you are the only one who somehow miraculously gets the address and zip code. I knew that to tell you my fantasies would probably make you happy, but I couldn't. First because I knew my fantasies were outrageous, but mostly they were a little trumped up and that I myself was sensationalizing it, maybe even fabricating it to fill the void in session. But the simple feeling was just that you are always there anyway. Probably the pressure too of having to see a total stranger doctor the next day and show him my womb—having to be jolly and open for him—yuk. Gynecologists are a whole different ballgame.

I waited six days to write this. It's the last time I will do it this way. From now on I will be serious.

In your write-ups you call me Ginny. Whereas I just talk to you. But maybe because of that I have to be more careful what I say, yours is a diary and mine's just a phone conversation where I'm always conscious that I am connected to you and someone can eavesdrop.

III

Summer

(May 26–July 22)

DR. YALOM

THIS WAS the first interview after Ginny and I had a chance to read each other's write-ups. I have looked forward to today with some trepidation. Primarily, I wondered if certain parts of what I had written might have an adverse effect on Ginny. In addition, I felt personally embarrassed after reading both sets of reports—some of my observations seemed sophomorish and my language ungainly in comparison to hers. One saving grace, though, was the fact that my accounts contained nothing but positive feelings toward her, since that's how I genuinely feel. At any rate, she came in rather bubbly. I suggested we tape-record this session in case we want to come back to it later. She said perhaps I should listen to the first few minutes of it, since I would probably be disappointed and change my mind about recording. She then went on to explain how a number of catastrophies had beset her since our last meeting: scabies, vaginal fungus disease, laceration of her foot, huge doctors' bills, and then finally the fact that Karl had not been out of the house much that week so that she had been obliged to read my reports hastily and her own scarcely at all.

Her initial response (not an unexpected one) was to compare her work unfavorably with mine. She felt as if she had taken a course, as it were, and turned in a poor term paper. She said that by comparison with mine, her papers looked puny and brief, whereas I had been willing to delve into things more deeply. She pointed out that my writing them in the third person, talking about Ginny, gave me a great deal more freedom than she had because she wrote them to me and used the pronoun "you." This observation really struck me because I hadn't noticed it before; it is so illustrative of the inequality of the psychotherapeutic relationship in general. I would never have considered writing them to "you." And what about her addressing me as "Dr. Yalom" and my calling her "Ginny"? Will it ever be comfortable for her to call me by my first name?

For the most part, her feelings about the reports were positive; in fact she said they had given her so much encouragement that she has decided not to take a full-time job, which would have forced her to discontinue therapy. I mused about what aspects of my writing had caused this reaction, but she simply replied that she now felt ready to move on to the second phase of her relationship with me. Recalling some of her past teachers, she noted that when they got around to giving her a symbolic testimonial dinner, it usually signified the end of the relationship. In one sense, these write-ups were a testimonial dinner. She apparently read them very quickly, focusing on all the positive aspects, and came away with the feeling that she doesn't have to worry so much about winning me over and can go on to other stages with me. She made quite an issue of the fact that she had no time to consume them carefully because she couldn't possibly read them around Karl, they were so incriminating. She made me feel as if we were conspirators in a political plot or lovers having an affair which had to be totally concealed from Karl. Obviously there is a grain of truth in this because if Karl were to read everything she has said about him, he might object to the mere fact that she was so public with their private life. Though I think that's the sum total of the possible offense he could take. It is clear that she over reacts to the threat of discovery; the secretiveness of it all, the careful concealment of the write-ups in her room, the pumping of her heart when she furtively reads them lest Karl come in and catch her at it.

The interview in general was rather nonproductive, aside from our sharing with one another our reactions to the write-ups. Ginny was pleased to talk about her ease in performing acts which had previously seemed major obstacles. For example, in the past when the kitchen was in shambles, she would bemoan the fact that the table was untidy and that she was the kind of person who made such a mess. Now she finds, almost in wonderment, that she can make the table tidy by rapidly cleaning it up.

We talked about money. Humiliation is her shadow: it is there when she begs her landlord to fix the hot water heater, when she asks for free medical care at the peoples' clinic and when she dons her outfit for her job as a traffic guard for school children, all the while praying silently that none of her friends will see her. She has a deeply engrained sense of herself as a demeaned person. I tried to help her see that she is the demeaner and that if she wants to be proud of herself, she has to do things in which she can take pride. So much of her aggravation stems from the lack of money in her life, a problem with a relatively easy remedy. I asked if she had seriously thought of putting her writing talent to work. There I was again preaching my personal gospel and without even a helpful text, since I had no concrete suggestions to add to the expression of my confidence in her ability to find a way to earn money in a manner appropriate to her talents.

May 26

GINNY

HE WANTED to record. I didn't bother to think about that or ask why. I didn't let it affect me as I went on humiliating myself by enumerating my diseases which were not crucial to anything but then were recorded to be played back. We were like Dick Cavett and his guest.

I talked about the General Practitioner and how I thought he was overcharging me. I sort of wanted to ask your professional advice, but I still felt unsettled after we'd talked about it. Maybe because talking is not acting. This morning I was awakened by dreams of confronting him. Mostly I trust everybody since I am too dependent not to. I react to someone rather than act first. They put me in a place, set my borders and limits. If they are bad, my stamina usually holds on longer than they do till they have passed. But this one doctor kept getting in deeper to my nightmares. Mostly because I have been getting cut up and infected. You are never a bad doctor in my dreams, only once when I was sure you did not like my encounter group leader, M. J., and I knew how wrong you were because your background and philosophy could not come to terms with his magic and psychodrama, however short-lived.

Maybe as a result of reading the write-ups, I experienced sensory dreams, in which I was bracketing and gliding, back and forth. I'm sure these reflect happiness somewhere.

In talking about the write-ups I breezed over them too much.

You were covering your face and removing your eyeglasses. And laughing in a way half-startled and shocked, and I knew you were, but I wasn't sensitive to it. You had given a lot more in the write-ups than I had, told a lot more. And I kind of cantered over it all without thanking you. In my mind I could do that because I promised myself *next* week I would look at them more closely.

I think I slur my words when I talk to you. I drop g's sometimes. Just to feel sloppier.

Even though I'm always saying how much I want to repay you, sometimes I know what you want and deliberately don't give it, staring at your shoe or the table. You want me to speak freer and to begin not to hold back thoughts, but it doesn't look like I'll let myself be broken of the habit. I take no responsibility for what I say, maybe that's why my write-ups are not as full as yours.

In the session I knew I was optimistic, but that's because I was removed from actual challenges and felt comfortable. We were talking about what I would do *next week,* not what I had to do then. I can be very happy when I imagine things that are not on my back yet.

Yesterday I told you how I would have to start doing things. You usually tell me. The focal point was the kitchen table. My training ground. But it was a revelation the first time I realized there was a path. How I could conquer trivia, not let it mount up against me.

By putting things off, I suspend my active life. Then when I am most passive, most of the things I haven't done and all the things that I have put a "hold" on, spin around, swirl in an inertia. Sometimes I like therapy because I feel it is a perfectly safe time. When I have only to prepare to do something but don't have to do it yet.

I know that Karl hates my inertia, my backing away, my production numbers. I hate it too but am kind of stuck. I do a lot of things with energy but seem to stop just short of perfection and a goal. In this way the kitchen table becomes like a great mesa with dust and tumbleweed that blows against me, no matter how much I straighten up. I know my problem has something to do with suspension of action and feeling. Sometimes I am terribly nervous. Something in me wants to do something. My desires are like a horse at the starting gate, that moment suspended, the red flag up, the horse straining and tense. If the horse is pulled back and strains too much within the gate, when the gates finally open and the race begins, he will relax all his tension and run the race badly, or at least have a bad start. The jockey has to know when to restrain and tense the horse, only seconds before the gates open so he will run with speed. Sitting in the waiting room, waiting for you, I tense up. Most times by the time I get to your office I'm just glad to be out of the starting gate, out of my tension, and run a slow race for both of us.

June 2

DR. YALOM

A VERY important, puzzling hour with Ginny. The kind of hour I would have expected last week. She began by saying that right after our last hour she mailed out several things she had written to *Mademoiselle.* Then she told me that over the weekend she had had a terrible panic during which she lay awake all night. She explained this on the basis of her yeast infection—she and Karl tried to have intercourse but she was very tight, it was "as though her vagina were sewn together." In the morning he asked her what was wrong and she told him some of the things we had talked about months ago—that she would appreciate it if he would make love to her longer, which might enable her to get more satisfaction. That following night they tried again and failed, which caused her to become very tense and upset, and lie awake all night, fantasying that Karl would leave her and all the while hoping he wouldn't hear the loud internal echo of her imaginary conversations with me. Again, she portrayed herself as the child or the slave in relation to Karl, wondering what he was feeling and what she might do for him and what he might like her to do, without ever a thought of the reciprocal perspective.

Very quickly she added in passing that she had reread the write-ups and in fact had started reading them before she went to bed on the night of the panic attack. She jokingly said that since then she doesn't read them at night anymore, only during the morning or day. This sounded to me as if it were terribly important, and we spent, needless to say, the rest of the hour on it.

To my mind I made heroic efforts to track down Ginny's reactions to my reports. She was incredibly resistive. I have not seen her quite so explicitly resistive to any issue in all the time I have known her. When I asked her about the write-ups, I had to cut through several layers of debris before we got into anything that was close to her feelings. She would start off with, "Well, I smiled when I read such and such," or "I felt that I was not being genuine or didn't take responsibility for asking such and such in a session." I kept pressing her to share with me her reactions to the revelations about me she had found in the reports. Surely she knows some things now that she hadn't known before, how did that make her feel? She avoided this on several occasions. I practically had to get her up against the wall and pin her arms behind her to make her talk. Some of the things she finally mentioned were exactly the ones I had felt most sensitive about writing, i.e., my borrowing phrases or techniques which I had read or heard from other psychiatrists and "using them" in my work with her; my hoping that she would see certain books in my office to make her think me better read; the innuendoes that I had worked on some problems similar to hers in my own therapy; my sexual or lack of sexual feelings toward her, which made her feel "squeamish." When we pursued the meaning of the word "squeamish," we didn't get anywhere, except that she felt it was like "getting a love letter from an older boy" which she used to read with her mother when she was younger.

She felt ashamed of evoking any feelings in me. She said she wasn't worth it, that she wasn't really "large enough," she wanted to be invisible. On a couple of occasions she said, "If only you could have seen me that night when I was panicked." I tried to find out what she would have wanted me to do that night, or what she could have expected from me, especially in the light of my reports, which disclose how fallible I am. She couldn't answer that except to say that she likes to be with someone when she is troubled, like her father or mother, when they would take her into their bed. I wondered aloud whether she was upset at the loss of my "perfection." She denied that, although at one point she mentioned that when she was leafing through the notes trying to restore her memory, she had a sudden impulse just to throw them on the floor in a dramatic flair. On another occasion toward the end of the hour she said something which suggested she was angry because I was so much in her mind whereas she was so little in mine. This startled me. It was quite the opposite of what she usually says—usually she presents herself as so lacking in importance that she doesn't deserve any regard at all. I think that her desire to be the sole recipient of my attention is the primary feeling. And the other feeling, of being so small or insignificant, is really a way of compensating for her sense of greed.

I felt very sorry that I hadn't tape-recorded this session. It's difficult for me, even now immediately afterwards, to capture its flavor, and I would like to be able to go over it. Naturally, I am concerned that the reports have made her feel somewhat badly. On another level, though, I have no doubt at all that they will hasten our work. When she said that it sounded as if I had worked on some similar problems in my own therapy, I said I had and asked how that made her feel. She evaded the question. Unfortunately I have to teach a class now and must end this report knowing I have captured only a small fragment of the hour.

June 2

GINNY

YOU'RE RIGHT. I don't want to write this. I feel like I gave away a friend by giving you back those write-ups. And a friend who only had stayed for a short visit. At the same time I was relieved that the occasion was past. I say I want them back sometime to look at and concentrate on, but that may be just my "I'll cry tomorrow" alibi. The part that made me cringe and which I remember just now is when you talked about my self-pitying cycle and getting sucked into it. That's seeing me as a lump.

The writings are horribly incriminating of me. I don't believe I am totally the way I am described by myself or you. Karl would surely leave me in a minute if it were true. And yet I nurture the "poor me" of the reports, supply transportation for it to come here each week, and keep away the less familiar stronger elements in me. It's easier to be stomped on than be the one who stomps.

I'm sitting here trying to fantasize you saying, "You know I like you Ginny." Then I get squeamish and say, "You idiot." But I can't go farther.

The bad night was not the focal point of the week, so I wonder why it became the only thing we talked about in session. I should have stopped it.

When I came into session I felt calm and open. But I put myself back into last Sunday night, like jumping into a well where you have once been caught. I started to explain the situation—it happened like this, see—and suddenly I'm right back where I started.

Yesterday when I left I realized there was nothing you could write in the write-ups or I could write that would magically change what didn't happen and give it sense. I know you feel sucked in, now that I've read your comments. But I can't come to a conclusion with *words* out loud. I never have. We nibble on little bait, a real fish is way below. The small things we catch, I throw back.

I know the only way we have of getting at anything is talking. But I get so self-conscious. I felt very bad about the session because I hadn't concentrated the way you wanted or on what you wanted. If we had been meeting twice a week, I could have jumped in again. Maybe I wouldn't though. I meet Karl every night and postpone things with a promise to work on our lives.

But I think you and I still want different things. I want to be mellow and calm and cry, and you want rational answers and leadership qualities.

The rest of the day should have been bad and discouraging but I didn't allow that. I wanted to erase and reverse the day and not follow my visions full circle, and I didn't.

June 11

DR. YALOM

FOR ME this was one of the least involved, least tangible meetings I have had with Ginny. As soon as she left my office, she left my mind, and now some four hours later, I can scarcely remember the interview; only that I had a strong sense of lack of work, lack of movement.

The most striking part of the session was the very beginning when Ginny hurled two tiny Ginny bolts at me. First she said it seemed over the phone (when she called to change the appointment) that I hadn't really wanted to see her this week. Then she added that she was a little ambivalent about coming today since she could have gone to the races instead and this is the last day of the season.

For some period of time then she talked about her depression, about her discouragement, about the fact that the last meeting had been a very bad one in which I was pressing her for some type of answer which she did not know and could not produce. (In fact, this was very much the case, since last session I spent most of the time trying to navigate her into the area of her feelings on reading the notes.) I made a couple of tenuous attempts in this session to pursue that question but it doesn't seem as if we'll be talking about the reports for quite some time.

She then told me how she habitually makes inventories of all the bad things about herself. I, for want of a more original tact, prodded her to mention some of the good things that had occurred this week. Well, she had tried out for a theatrical group and had written a funny poker form for some of her friends, which proved to be hilarious but without commercial value. In response to my interest in her acting, she told me that she sometimes acted through her mother, by asking her mother to portray a scene, which she could then mimic perfectly. She has thought of being a professional actress and apparently has considerable talent. She couldn't really own that and began to go through some subtle and elaborate moves to undermine whatever positive thoughts she may have let slip out. For example, after admitting that she acts pretty well, she immediately added that she is simply putting on an act, i.e., not really feeling the feelings in the way that she should. It does get very wearying for me and at times I feel as if I've exhausted my inventiveness in encouraging Ginny to look at herself in a different way.

And so we ended without really having said "hello" today. The only hopeful signs were some flickerings of rebellion, for example, her initial comment that she believed I had not wanted to see her today. Oh, yes, also she arrived some fifteen minutes late, having taken a bus which could not possibly have gotten her here on time. Furthermore she was somewhat directive in recalling a dream she had last night: "I'll tell you about it, but I don't want to spend much time talking about it." The dream was that I couldn't see her in individual therapy, but that I did allow her to sit in on one of my classes. In that class I wrote a few words on the board, which she wrote down in her notebook. It was some type of psychological jargon, like names of various diseases. Then, feeling sorry for her, I saw her privately for ten to fifteen minutes. The fact that we were both writing things down, I on the blackboard, she in her notebook, brought to my mind the whole issue of the write-ups. The dream (and her initial comments) reflect her fear that I do not wish to see her but underneath this surface concern I sense the first delicate blades of her overt resistance to therapy.

June 11

GINNY

I EXPECTED to be disappointed with last Friday's therapy. Instead when I left I felt better. But this is Monday and only certain things stand out in my mind.

First, when we talked about my crying over Lassie. I thought it was a bad thing, an example of a childish emotional mentality. But you said some people could not even do that. This rejuvenated me, because it was something I hadn't thought of, except in a satiric light. Karl vomits when he catches me with the last five minutes of *Lassie*.

I think when we counted up plusses, I was roping you in. It's like remembering plots of a novel never written. The plusses are very far removed if they cannot sustain me and motivate me. And they are dry to go over.

When you thought I was being phoney, I enjoyed that. I think I'm always so sincere even to my own dullness. It must have really been bad, uncomfortable for you, if you thought I was phoney.

I came away from the session optimistic. Though I sensed that you did not enjoy it. But that didn't detract from my pleasure.

June 15

DR. YALOM

ROUND 3 (or is it Round 4 or 5) in the Ginny get angry series. I put so much pressure on Ginny today, I can't believe it myself, and I wonder what she'll do this time and how many more times we'll have to go through the cycle.

It all began when she walked into my office crest-fallen and depressed saying, "We had another 'lump' talk last night." (She was referring to an earlier conversation when Karl had accused her of being a sexual lump). The gist of this talk was that Karl had relentlessly criticized her because of her many failures—a criticism she considered justified on his part. He was asking for some interaction with her, for some kind of spontaneity, and everything he said about her was "absolutely true." She couldn't respond to him or responded as though she were someone else sans emotions. It was a total nightmare, she just waited until it was over so that she could be mercifully relieved from everything. Since then she's been besieged with fantasies of his leaving her and she thought for sure that "this was it." She comes to me today in a very self-critical, self-deprecating mood and I knew if I were to spin around with her for awhile, I would be sucked into her despair and self-disgust. It was important to-day to think first and feel second.

My first response was to try and find out what she would have said to Karl had she not been so paralyzed. She couldn't really come up with anything, except to say that a "real woman" might have stuck up for herself a bit more. Several of her statements implied that she must have been sitting on considerable indignation and anger but couldn't come to terms with these emotions.

A review of last night's chronology clarified what had happened. The scenario went like this. Ginny spent from 5:00 to 7:00 trying to cook a new dish, roast pork loin. The meal was a semi-failure, edible but not interesting. Karl, who reads during his dinner anyway, read a crossword puzzle all through the meal and criticized her as if she were a waitress, saying the pork was poor and the potatoes were not done, etc. Following dinner he was to have taken her to a friend's so she could get a shower. (She can't shower at home because there is still brown water coming in from the tap which somehow has never been fixed.) He refused to drive her over to Eve's, obliging her to take a streetcar. Following that, when she came home he was gone, leaving a note that he had gone out to have some beers and hoping that he would get over his bad mood. She was relieved by the note. When he came back he was probably even more upset because she hadn't acknowledged the note. He sat watching television a little bit and then shortly after 12:30 they turned off the set and she was asleep in a few minutes. Ginny says that since she gets up at 6:30 in the morning, she becomes very tired by midnight. In any event, Karl was angry with her for falling asleep so early.

From this point on in the interview, I came down extremely hard on Karl and very consciously too. What I wanted to do was to turn Ginny on her head and for once help her stop thinking of all the things that Karl finds unsatisfactory in her, so that she will stop living in the shadow of fear of his sudden desertion. I wanted her to enter-tain the thought that Karl has certain severe flaws, and thus I said to her, "How long are you going to give Karl to straighten up?" I pointed out as clearly as I could that she turns off anytime she has any anger. She can express anger only passively, for example by not cleaning the house, or by not clearing all the clothes off the chair. She replies she's never been able to clean the house. I said I thought that was ridiculous and that she could do it anytime she wanted to, but doesn't, as a means of expressing her anger. That's what we call passive-aggressive. At this point she suddenly burst out crying and expressed the wish that she were a five-year-old child again, where she wouldn't have to worry about doing anything for anybody. I pressed on into the subject of Karl's flaws, supplying many leads along the way. We got to such things as his lack of intuition, his lack of sensitivity to her, his constant reading, especially at meals, his need to control which is so oppressive that her friend Eve doesn't like to have him around. He criticizes her, she said, because she's not growing, not improving her abilities. I asked her if reading crossword puzzles all the time and doping out races can be construed as self-improvement. It doesn't seem as if he's been growing either. We talked, or I talked, about his lack of generosity, the fact that he still charges her money for the tolls on bridges, whereas he can earn $40 a day whenever he pleases to work. I told her that I think the response of almost any other woman to his dinner criticism would have been, "Who the hell are you to criticize me?" I kept saying to Ginny, "Is this the kind of man you want to live with?" while she responded that she won't have to because sooner or later he'll leave her. I kept pressing her with the question, "Do you want to spend the rest of your life with a person like this? If not, how much longer are you going to give him to change?" I wondered about the possibility that she is also depriving him of any chance to grow because she never gives him any feedback, and I'm sure that that was what some of the fuss was about last night. She cried a couple more times during the session. We talked about his lack of praise for any of her virtues or talents. He doesn't say anything about her writing or about her clever parodies or about her acting; wouldn't another woman want and expect some positive response to these things?

She heard me giving her some explicit instructions and asked somewhat tremulously if she has to do it right away since they have an important poker game at their house in three days. I honestly feel that if I had told her to go home and tell Karl to fuck off, she might well have done it this very day. She pointed out, however, that it would seem forced. Of course, that's part of the real danger that I face with Ginny: she's so passive, so puppet-like, she'll do exactly as I tell her to do, which may not help her feel totally autonomous in the long run. Well, screw it, that's just one of the risks we'll have to take. I think I'm beginning to feel we ought to work with behavior first, feeling later. At any rate, I was extremely indelicate and rather powerful during the meeting, in that I didn't even allow Ginny to tell me how she felt I was coming across. I don't know what she'll do with this, but in the past it's been this kind of session which she's most appreciated.

June 15

GINNY

THE SESSION gave me a lot of information and some strength. Whenever this happens, I always wonder—what would I do without you and the session?

I felt I was really there. At the same time I didn't care how I was affecting you, for once. At the end I knew I was exasperating you, but that didn't bother me either, although I felt a little tired from being so tepid.

Before the session I had been so much in a fantasy. This is how I deal with things. Fantasy is resilient. I had no expectations about the session. I went into it blind. I was fantasying so much I didn't even think about the session. I wasn't even going to bring up the night before since it seemed so obvious. Of course I was glad when I did, and once I did, I don't think I backed away from myself except toward the end.

Your word "indignation" sent up sparks in me. Once my father was playing with me but took a nickel I knew was rightfully mine (just a small thing). I wanted it back; he was teasing me, and when he finally gave it to me, I started crying. Maybe because I felt so sorry for all the bad things I had inside, indignation. Karl teases too all the time. I would rather think nothing than think something bad of someone. Suspend judgment and everything. I don't think you're going to get me to express bad thoughts about people, though I would like to try. I'm from the school of Bambi—Don't say anything at all if you can't say something good.

I could hear your voice all throughout the session, by friction, trying to catch my voice and give it some fire. I kept resisting, as your voice grated more and more on my ears. I felt hostile to you. That you were trying to manipulate me. And wanted me at least to mimic you in ferocity.

But the change in me afterwards was incredible. I realize that any anger or friction in my life paralyzes me. I dread it. I lay quiet and restless and tense at night waiting for it, that anger ambush. I fear any confrontation. But now (or at least for three hours after the session) I have been welcoming it. I waited for it. As an opportunity to expand myself and find myself. (Karl was almost too nice to me. Why didn't he do something characteristic—insult my hamburgers—so I could let loose and haul one at him?) I felt more alive because I wasn't waiting in fear to go empty and blank at the first sign of trouble. I felt larger than myself, rather than smaller. More surprises happened. And for a few days afterwards I didn't fantasize, for what was all around me felt pleasant and powerful. I also didn't write the write-up completely because when we have a good session, what has happened seems to evade words and to be still happening.

Of course, I have fantasied since then, dreaded since then, and procrastinated a lot. I need more than one jolt. But even that small push you gave me allows me to coast for awhile, free from fear and full of feeling. That is wonderful. Why don't you scream a little more?

June 23

DR. YALOM

THINGS ARE rather gay and silly and bilaterally coquettish. There was an obvious disparity between Ginny's demeanor and the content of her talk. Her content was "down"—she was desperately hoping I could do today what I did last week; her demeanor was high-spirited. She wore a rather absurd costume with Farmer John clodhoppers and overalls. During the interview she said she felt somewhat awkward about the shoes, but that she blistered whenever she wore any other kind. Last time she had wanted to look nice and had worn another pair, but her feet blistered. I didn't pick up her comment about wanting to look nice the last time, but perhaps I should have.

Her main message was that what we had done last time was very helpful to her. She had had a different attitudinal set all week, especially in regard to Karl. It wasn't so much that she had the opportunity to answer him back, but that she was set to do so should he torment her in any way. It seems as if her set conveyed something to Karl, so that he was quite different during the week and in fact more self-critical than she's noted in the past. For example, he would say "What a slob I've been," or "Look at the mess I left at the table." Once or twice she actually did stick up for herself. But she knew she could never fight back if Karl were to make some sort of sexual insult. I tried to push her into what kind of insult that might be. She said, well he might accuse her of faking orgasm. I wondered then what she might say to him in return. (I wanted her to know that, though I don't advise this kind of sexual insult between couples as a good way of fighting, if it came to that, she too had some ammunition with which to fight back.) I was merely trying to bring her to the point of realizing that she has as much right as he has to attack unfairly.

On another matter she refused the right to have judgments about people. She spoke of her sister who is very judgmental of her, but she, Ginny, cannot bring herself to respond in kind. Finally I was obliged to act as Ginny's mouthpiece, to say that her sister is pretentious and sometimes acts like an ass, and to instruct Ginny to say these things after me. In the midst of our discussion about the sister and about Karl, Ginny interrupted to say, "I wish we could do what we did last time." I found this very odd since I thought I was doing just that. I think she says "do it" and "don't do it" in the same breath.

In general, though, Ginny is right. Active instruction in the art of aggression is perhaps the best thing for her now; if we can do this for several weeks in a row, then it will probably permanently change her feelings about herself. Yet I shy away from becoming so authoritarian because I fear that will only enhance her dependency; my telling her to be aggressive still conveys the message of submission to me. It is also clear that she can't follow me for more than a week at a time.

Nevertheless, she had a good week, she even won money at poker, and it was only in the last couple of days that she started going down again. Going down means that she's spent the last two days in day-dreaming, as was the case the entire week prior to our last meeting. She intimated at the beginning of the interview that what she's really not doing is writing. What difference does it make if she stands up to Karl about doing the dishes, the important thing is that she is not writing. She *had* written something last night that she wanted me to see and was sorry she hadn't typed it up, but it had something critical of Karl, which stopped her from typing in his presence; she'll bring it in in the future. She is still with the acting group, doing improvisations in the evenings, and may well get a job with them in the fall. It is incredible for me to think of her as willing and eager to act *à l'improviste*—one of the most terrifying of all situations—I would no sooner do that than parachute into Mt. Etna. I have a hard time reconciling it with the picture of Ginny as "timid" and "frightened."

I spent the last part of the interview focusing on the writing, not with great inventiveness. What would it take to make her start writing? What is she writing? What is she not writing? I tried to push her into thinking about tomorrow; what would her schedule be? Could she start writing at 10:00, if she wanted to? I tried to determine what would mobilize her will. She got angry at this, responding with genuine irritation, and I was taken aback. Now ten minutes later I can reflect almost with pleasure on the fact that she was able to do this. She said that she thinks she will write tomorrow and will start at 10:00 o'clock. I ended the session by jotting down on a piece of paper "Write at 10:00 a.m.," folded it up and gave it to her. She jokingly said she would pin it on her blouse. It is kind of a joke as she sees it, but I'm dead serious and have a hunch we'll be hearing more about that piece of paper. I feel rather enthusiastic, optimistic, definitely high today after seeing Ginny. It was an exciting hour and she was really quite charming. She told me a couple of jokes, funny things that she had done during the week, and I got a much clearer sense than ever before of how much fun it must be for Karl to live with her. Obviously I've known this intellectually for quite some time, but rarely see the jaunty, witty side.

June 23

GINNY

I NEVER really got to deep feelings. I have been dawdling. As you said, the real issue is writing. When you kept nagging me about why I wasn't writing, I had to form an answer and mumble it out; I guess I could have gotten angry. Because I felt bugged, because it sounded like my parents trying to coax my "gifts" into something constructive. And obviously these apparent talents are encrusted with something else that makes them hard to mine. But I always feel I have to answer. I'm strung out on "I'm going to's."

I phased out today, like when you're saying the obvious about writing or making judgments. I pretend to listen to you and go along with you, keeping up my side of the conversation when really I don't take any of it personally or seriously. So I want you to change the subject but I do this by grinning rather than saying I'm bored.

On the way home in the bus I fell asleep and woke up with a start, dismayed, to realize the session was over. It wasn't a bad session. It's like ordering the wrong thing in a restaurant. You've missed your chance till next time and have to digest what you've eaten.

It always seems that the follow-up session after a good session is poor in comparison. Cause I know that the one before injected me with new strength and purpose. Whereas last time I just came and was my unchanging self—a butterfly under glass. And I think it's a ruse to talk about my muse (no!) to talk about my writing. If there's one thing worse than going back to my past, which I know you don't like from reading your write-ups, its going into my future. It's true, if I were writing, or if I could stand up for myself and not feel ashamed of separating myself from other people by judgments or emotions, the therapy and I would be improved. For instance, I think that there are things in Karl I really don't like, mean silent things that are not all of him. But I stop in front of the bad things and go dead in sadness and talk about my bad things instead. Why can't I just tell him and myself what I don't like, what's wrong, what should be thrown out, given up to Goodwill and then we could move on realistically, and I wouldn't feel ashamed or incriminating. I'd just be growing and so would he. If I could only admit there are some things I don't like about Karl, and other things I love, then I wouldn't try to kill it all.

Just as you want these write-ups to be about what happens in the session, I think the session should stick to what I am doing. It seems like I am living in an 'if' clause in therapy; my life dangling from a hanging if. Because when we talk about writing, or what I might write, I gloss and glide with optimism and not till I get home and the 10 o'clock hour comes and I start sticking pins into myself or turn into Mrs. Slothman, do I realize it was an impersonation of myself that came to Palo Alto and buzzed for an hour with someone like my father who knows I'd be all right if I just wrote.

Of course I've left this write-up till too late, so only general impressions of the session and myself are remembered or induced.

I really wanted to read you last week what I had written in my journal from the night before and what I kept alluding to. At least then you could have heard that side of me. And maybe you would have seen how self-indulgent and easy it was.

June 30

DR. YALOM

IN GENERAL my feeling is that I've wasted an hour and Ginny, I guess, has wasted several hours. It takes her three or four hours to get the bus, walk here from the station and then go back. Although of course I try to rationalize my sense of wasted time. What do I tell

students? Oh yes, it's time spent "strengthening the relationship."
Therapy is a slow construction project, requiring months and years,
one can't expect something tangible from each hour—there are hours
of frustration that you and the patient have to sit through together.
If the therapist requires and expects personal gratification from every
therapy hour, he will either go mad himself or move into a crash
program of break-through psychotherapy, like primal screaming, a
form of madness itself. The mature therapist moves deliberately and
patiently, that's what I tell my students and that's what I tell myself
today. But there are times when it is difficult to maintain the faith.
At any rate, things started off by her telling me that she was in a very
bad mood, she had lost her wallet a couple of days ago and had just
learned about it today. She had had a bad ride down. She had been
approached sexually by a fifteen-year-old boy when she was lying out
in the park before our session and, furthermore, she hadn't been able
to tell him off! She had lost $3.00 at a poker game in the first hour of
play and then retired to her bedroom and pouted and sulked while
the game continued for at least another four hours. She had had
several job interviews, without success and so forth.

I hardly knew where to start. The common thread in everything
she said was some dimly perceived anger. For a moment I let my own
fantasy play and the smoky image that came to mind was a huge
lava bed with bubbles coming up and puffs of anger exploding to the
surface and Ginny being confused and overwhelmed by it all. I decided to investigate all of these incidents, so that Ginny would
recognize and possibly re-experience the trail of her anger.

I was also most curious as to whether my "Write at 10 a.m." note
had had any effect. Ginny said she had written yesterday and the
day before (with no mention of the rest of the week). She tended to
negate her accomplishments by pointing out that she had been able
to write for only an hour and a half, although seven pages were com-
pleted during this time. I baited her by nagging about the writing.
Why hadn't she written last week? Why doesn't she write continuously? I suspected if I nagged enough, we'd see some anger surface
at me.

Then we did things like talking about the poker game and her
anger at a friend who came late, whom Ginny publicly defended on
the grounds that she was baking cookies, which made Ginny feel like
a fool when the friend arrived cookie-less; her anger at having lost so

much money so fast; her anger at one of her male friends who broke a door, which made Ginny fear the landlord would kick them out; her anger at everyone for staying all night and the feeling that the landlord would dislike their harboring so many great drunken types; her rage then at the little boy who made a sexual advance toward her, and her furor at herself for not being able to say something like "beat it" or, "get out of here, you creep." Instead she merely picked herself up and walked away, saying good-bye and thinking of what her friends might have said to him. Of course, then she looked at the other side and thought how badly that would have made this fifteen-year-old feel. Then she talked about her anger at me, especially how she would feel at the end of the hour. I tried to get her to pretend it was the end of the hour, four o'clock instead of three-thirty. What were some of the things she would then like to say to me? She gave this only a token try. I continued to push her more about the writing and she almost flared up, but said only "O.K., O.K., I'll write." What she didn't say was "for Christ's sake, get off my back." I said that for her and she smiled wanly. It looks as though her patience is finally being tried and I think it is a good thing—how long have I been pushing her to feel and express her anger?

In any event, we both left with a vague unsatisfied feeling. I spent some time asking her to look at the bright, positive side of her life. Though everything seems black to her today, the situation with Karl is surely much improved. She's quite convinced now that he really loves her. She's able to answer him back on several issues. Somehow or other, things have gotten freed up for her sexually. She is writing, she is not lonely, she has several friends, and I insisted that these things are much closer to the core of Ginny than the trivial items she had mentioned. Her response to this was that she had told me at the start of the session that these were trivial items. Here again, she was close to being angry with me and I phrased her anger for her. "It was stupid for me to have said that since you already said it at the beginning of the hour." Ginny sort of smiled again, in tacit acknowledgement. As I dictate this interview it begins to sound better than the way I experienced it during the passage of the hour.

June 30

GINNY

I FELT cocky and giddy, but wanted to feel sad and truthful. (You would say—Ginny, find other words, the bright side of cocky and giddy.) My anger makes me feel both alive and dead. I'm right in the middle of it with an upset stomach. The more aware of the feeling of anger I am, the more spunk I have. Then something inside of me throws a blanket over my head. And I kind of walk around without direction but in a general frenzy.

At the end of the hour, when you said 4:20 was actually a better time for you to meet, you showed just enough mundane assertiveness to give me an example of a person standing up for what he wants. I like to see you strong and reacting just like an ordinary person. Somehow I learn from these encounters, however trivial.

Again I felt entertaining today but I didn't bother to question if you wanted to be entertained. I should ask if that gets us anywhere rather than just barrel along under my own nervousness.

How do I get into deeper thoughts? You said at the end that things were going fairly well in my life but that I was only bringing up the petty things.

I can't concentrate with you on things you want me to think about. I remove myself from the person you are speaking to.

July 12

DR. YALOM

LAST WEEK I missed my interview with Ginny. I had two colleagues in town most of the week, we were working day and night on a book on encounter groups, and I started cancelling out

100

most of my appointments when I saw that we wouldn't be able to finish what we had to do. I called my secretary and told her to call Ginny to see whether she could possibly come in on Friday. My secretary misunderstood me and cancelled Ginny's appointment altogether, which was not what I had wanted. I later found out Ginny couldn't come in on Friday. Once I learned this, I tried to call Ginny at home to see if she could come in at some other time, but could not reach her. I was rather sorry that all this had happened but at the same time I knew that I was too swamped and too harassed to have been very effective in seeing her on Wednesday.

Ginny came in today and I explained what had happened to her. Her response to this was not even to acknowledge what I had said, but to tell me that she felt extremely depressed and had been now for some time; she used the word "bored" as well. The next thing she did was to ask me whether I had been at the movies last Monday, she thought she had seen me there. I told her that I hadn't. I then made an orthodox and, I think, accurate interpretation: it sounded to me as if she had some unstated feelings about my cancelling since she immediately talked about being depressed and then imagined she had seen me at the movies, hoping it was me so I could watch her behavior, watch her touch Karl, watch her eat popcorn, watch her drink coke, watch her eat Mound bars. This wish to see me more was, I think, created to deal with her hurt at my cancelling our time together. She denied all of this and laughingly suggested I had a good imagination, indeed I must be "writing a novel."

Then again in an extremely depressed tone she continued telling me how badly she had been feeling. Curiously some of the content of what she said seemed rather hopeful: she may have gotten a job which she really wanted, teaching English to foreigners at an adult education school. Though it looks certain, she won't know definitely for a couple of days. Since there was no obvious cause for her depression in any of the things that she brought up, I was convinced that my cancelling last week was important and decided to pursue it stubbornly today.

When she talked about her relationship to Karl, how uptight she felt and how unable she was to tell him she was feeling badly, I began thinking of the parallels between Karl and me. Whenever Ginny feels she had done the wrong thing with Karl, she fears he will throw her out, and the same with me. So I tried to help her say some of the things to me that she couldn't say either to Karl or to me. I continued to hone in very hard on her feelings about my missing last week. I kept saying to her that she was not really expressing her true feelings. She grew slightly impatient with this, but I persisted, and she went on to say that she felt just a bit of disappointment. I told her to take that little bit of disappointment and examine it through a magnifying glass and tell me what it looked like. She then admitted she had been sorry it was my secretary calling; couldn't I have called her myself? And she added that some of her friends who were at her place when my secretary called made fun of her for seeing a psychiatrist anyway; they say it is the psychiatrist who makes her feel bad and if she stopped seeing me, she'd be O.K. Mainly, she said, it was just a big bore not to have had something to do during the week I had cancelled.

We moved deeper and deeper into her feelings, and I said to her that she now has permission to ask me any question she wants. As she had all sorts of fantasies about last week, why didn't she check them out? So she asked me what I was doing last week and I told her. She then asked if I had any curiosity about what was happening to her. I told her that I did, which was true. I kept asking her to pose other questions which she really wanted to know. She felt blocked and could go no farther. I told her that I thought her depression was really a reaction to my not having seen her, that it probably had a long history and went back a long time in her life, and I thought she was really saying to me, "See what you've done to me," and that she depressed herself in an effort to punish me. She responded to this somewhat affirmatively. I wondered if she doesn't do something comparable with Karl. Then I tried to boggle her mind and change the frame by saying, "Your mission is accomplished, I do feel guilty and badly that I didn't see you last week and your being depressed has now worked. There is no further need for you to continue. Now let's go on to the next episode." She laughed at this. At one point early in the interview she did have the ability to say, "Can't you give me something, can't you give me some spark to get me out of this?" which is again an unusually hearty statement from Ginny.

I told her that I would feel so much closer to her if she could come into the interview and give me hell if she were upset about something that I did wrong, rather than coming in, sitting on her ass and pretending she was in a morgue, as a way of attempting to injure me for having hurt her. I told her I was sure the same thing was true with Karl and that if she felt put upon by the relationship, or if she felt the relationship was unsatisfactory in any way, she was deliberately insuring it would end by not opening up to Karl some of her feelings. By not talking about her pain, she puts herself even further from him, as she does from me.

July 12

GINNY

YOU ARE too intellectual sometimes and encourage my own far-fetched analogies. Like when you asked how I felt about missing the session. And because I didn't see you then, isn't that why I thought I saw you in the movies? It's a kind of burlesque of psychiatry, like a script we are both writing. If I thought you were thinking like that, I'd know we were both just chatting meaninglessly.

I disliked the grin on my face whenever I answered one of your questions. It's like when I'm in upon myself, I'm grim with no expression. But as soon as you summon me, give me a lead and a chance to respond, I'm all giddy.

I liked the technique of putting a magnifying glass over a specific incident to try and etch out all the emotions. That's sort of putting life in slow motion. Which is what I like. Only I think the incident was not big enough. Actually there were two sides, or emotions, I felt. I gave you the one I thought you were prodding me for and wanted—that is, when you called, I was disappointed and a little angry. The other side of my miser's coin is that I was relieved—one trip less. Save $2.00, more time to do other things, and no Greyhound.

The only time I felt something in the session was when I hurt you, by suggesting I didn't care if I didn't see you. Then I felt guilty and sad. I felt removed from the self that is so off-hand, without emotions.

I was filled with hope and at the beginning of a new chapter when you said to try out my questions and needs on you before I risk them on K. "Try it out on me," you said. And that seemed like a great adventure.

But I'm always just browsing. At the end of the session, though, I was revived. No matter how I'm feeling, I can be thoroughly revived, just by attention. I liked your theory that as a way of getting even I become dead and more depressed and succeed in making others feel guilty and your conclusion that since I'd done it, now I could move on to something new. When you gave me the article on Hemingway I had asked you about, that was a special prize.

I refuse though to take the individual beats, movements of the session seriously. Maybe that's why I can't succeed in the write-ups generalizing as I do, catching or slurring feelings, allowing them a few hours right after the session, and then ignoring them, or not thinking back on them in the week.

July 22

DR. YALOM

GINNY called today and asked if I could see her at 3:00 rather than at 4:00. As things worked out, that was convenient for me and I agreed. It was an unusual thing for her to do, just the kind of request she's usually afraid to make. She started the hour by saying she had been in a terrible stupor for the last two days, but before that had had an extremely good week. She obviously wanted to tell me about the bad period, but I couldn't help being a bit more curious about the good one. She said that something had happened in our last session which had been enormously relieving to her; it was my "Mission Accomplished" statement, that, through being depressed, she had succeeded in making me feel guilty and my candor in suggesting that she cash in her winnings on this maneuver and now devote her energies to something else. The importance of this is that I made something explicit which she was doing implicitly and thus stripped it of its strength because, to operate, it must remain unconscious.

This week's problem concerns the two-week course she is presently taking in order to teach English. She has, on two occasions, mispronounced Cuba (Cuber) because of her New York accent. The teacher has caught her at it and Ginny is strongly convinced she will fail the course, which could be a catastrophe of the greatest magnitude. I began to work on this problem by opening my huge grab-bag of various approaches and pitching them at her one after the other. Some of the approaches were reasonably robust, some were creaky old techniques that I rolled in on a wheelchair. I tried to help her understand that this was hardly a catastrophe which could change the course of her life in one way or another. I tried to point out that it was, in the long skein of her life, a relatively trivial event and something quite distant from the core of Ginny. I tried to make her think of things in the past which seemed tremendously important at the time, but now had been all but forgotten, so as to help her place this recent incident in a proper perspective. I wondered why she feels that the teacher had the right to define her totally and that if he flunked her out of the class, it would mean that Ginny is nothing. I even ironically proposed that she imagine her epitaph as reading, "Here lies Ginny, failed by Mr. Flood in the English-for-Foreigners Course." I tried another avenue of approach by suggesting that she may well be misperceiving the situation. It didn't seem too likely to me, as Ginny claims, that this teacher really wants to fail her so he can enjoy the exertion of power. I suggested that since she foresaw a possible failure, she could do something to head off the anticipated "calamity." Perhaps the teacher has not yet had the occasion to see some of Ginny's finer points; perhaps he might have an opportunity, as the class goes on, to appreciate certain strengths, such as her wit or tenacity. None of these approaches was very effective. There she was, ten years old in a crisply starched yellow dress, playing dodge ball, sticking her tongue out at me and neatly ducking every throw I made. I have a hunch, however, that by sheer intensity of effort I've done something to assuage her. Oh yes, another aspect we worked on was her feeling that Karl must have thought her stupid when she was unable to answer certain questions in the class (Karl is taking the course with her). I wondered if that could be possible, since it seems unlikely that Karl hasn't already learned to appreciate her intelligence after living with her so long.

Another subtheme in the interview was an article I had written with my wife on Ernest Hemingway which I gave her at the end of the last hour. One of the first things she said was that she had liked the article very much. Later she said that she hadn't understood I had written it with my wife. I suggested she ask me whatever she wished about my wife. She asked "What does she teach?" and I told her French and Humanities and then asked if there were anything else she wanted to know and she said, "No, that's all." All she would say was that she hadn't quite understood my wife was a professor too—she had seen her once on the street and now she thinks she must have met her in the University. I tried to pry up some other reactions, suspecting there were feelings of jealousy and sensing some tension, but she could not or would not continue.

One other theme was that she had had some fantasies last night of getting sicker and sicker and of Karl running away with some pretty girl he knew from his job, and that I would take Ginny away to some little cabin deep in the country, which was a kind of hospital run by one of my colleagues who was a good friend and who would help her get better by encouraging her to express anger and do all the things she can't do, and I would come and visit her there once in awhile. I pointed out to her, of course, that this fantasy arises in the wake of a very good week and that it seems dangerous for her to have too good a week, since it brought with it the threat of having to stop seeing me.

A last bit of self-criticism was Ginny's lament that she isn't "serious," that she's never serious about anything she does, that she tends to be too "flippant," even about therapy. I had a hard time understanding quite what she meant, as I see her as quite serious. Her flippancy and sense of humor are very much a part of her charm and I should hate for her to attempt to excise them surgically.*

---

* Tapes and notes for the next three meetings have been lost.

IV

A Passing Winter

(October 26–February 21)

DR. YALOM

IT HAS BEEN three months now since I have seen Ginny. I have been so busy I can't say that I thought of her or missed her a great deal, but I realized as soon as she came into my office that there is a kind of Ginny essence which clings to me.

As soon as I sat down and spent even five minutes with her, I was transported back to a different psychological place with old familiar terrain—a place I hadn't visited for many months. Ginny told me all the things she has been doing. She had a steady job for three months, working forty hours a week till she got laid off because of circumstances beyond her control. She has continued to live with Karl and things have gone well with them. She no longer dwells within the shadow of his immediate departure. They occasionally talk about going to South America with the understanding that they would go together, though she's not sure she really wants to leave the States. She's made new friends and talked to them instead of me, but she's also had many fantasy conversations with me in my absence. After this apparently "good report" she rested her case, and began to consider the "wicked" side of her existence. She feels she has not been living authentically but simply coasting along, smug and happy. I suggested she reconsider her definition of living—maybe her real living doesn't occur only in her tortured moments. She asked whether I was serious, whether this is what a psychiatrist considers progress. I told her she was afflicted with a disease of hyper-consciousness and she conceded that she has always watched herself too closely. She has been too much a part of the audience, too little a member of the cast.

With Karl the relationship has decidedly improved; yet Ginny feels strongly that she is not really relating to him, that she is not able to be profoundly "serious," and though she wants something different between them, she can't clearly explain what it is. When pressed, she said she wants Karl to look her in the face and say her name. They spend all their time together, daytime and nighttime. They work at the same job, both teaching in an adult education center, and I gather they are busy enough to work the whole day together without any particular strain. Nighttime is different, though, with the matter of sex still painfully unresolved. Ginny feels she should be more honest with Karl about her sexual inadequacy, that she should tell him everything, and I feel, though I do not say this to her, that there are some private subjects she should keep to herself. She wishes she could have an encounter group meeting with Karl where she could face him with her deepest fears, without his being able to pass them off lightly. I suggested to her, not completely in jest, that she bring him into the next session. She panicked at this and insisted that Karl doesn't believe in psychiatry.

At one point she said she's the same Ginny she was when she started therapy. I asked if she really believes that. When she repeated that she feels she is the same inside, I could not refrain from pointing out the changes I've seen in her. It is true, she admits, that her relationship with Karl has changed—he does fifty percent of the housework now, she doesn't have to pay for the gasoline in the car anymore—but she quickly takes away these gains from herself by saying that if it weren't for me, these things would never have happened. I tried to make her aware of her game, in which she disclaims all her winnings by allotting them to me. By the end of the session she was fairly angry with me and said that I was acting just like her parents when they tell her everything is going to be all right.

She also discussed her concern about my publishing her reports, which prompted me to ask if she remembered our agreement. She remembered I had promised not to publish them without her permission, and added that, since Karl knows who I am, under no circumstance could they ever be published under my name. And that includes even after her death. Jokingly, she said she wanted the movie rights as well. I must say, as she spoke, I felt disappointed. But she is perfectly right, though as time goes on, she may change her mind and feel differently about them or we'll both publish them anonymously. But we'll probably just forget them, because I don't think they are of the quality that warrants publication.

November 1

DR. YALOM

A RATHER strange, touching, truncated hour with many intriguing ebbs and flows.

I had a cast on my leg (a knee injury) and the office was all rearranged and disordered, and I sat in a different place and Ginny sat down and just started talking without commenting on the obvious. She's the first person I've seen who hasn't immediately asked about my leg. She started off by saying she felt like being silent today—let's just do something different. The first ten or fifteen minutes were quite strained. Ginny was obviously embarrassed and when she started talking I sensed a definite sexual undercurrent in everything she said. She said that Karl was disappointed she had returned to therapy, that he wished she would get so well she wouldn't have to see me anymore. Later she spoke of her inability to show me her feelings, adding that she doesn't show her feelings to either of us (me or Karl). Struck by her reference to "the two men" in her life, I asked if Karl responds to me as the "other man." Of course, she denied it. Later on she used the term "impregnable" in conveying her attitude toward both of us, and immediately the word "impregnable" evoked in me fantasies of pregnancy. She then went over the events of the past week, all of which suggested an unusually good period; she and Karl had gone down to Big Sur and things had gone very smoothly between them. She had a good time, but there is something missing in her life and she doesn't know what.

She told me a dream, though protesting it was unimportant. (Whenever I hear that, my ears perk up; it always means an important dream is coming.) Dream: There's a psychiatrist and a girl and the girl is very weird, does funny things with her hands. She's schizophrenic. The psychiatrist likes her a great deal, takes care of her for a long time, and then finally urges her to go away with a boy who returns from Viet Nam. The boy is a combination of her brother (in reality she has no brother) who went to Viet Nam to be killed, and another boy. At first things work out very nicely with the boy, but then he starts to be very mean to her, and she becomes more and more schizophrenic and ends by becoming catatonic. In the dream, before she and the boy move away, the psychiatrist teaches her how not to have children and also tells them not to go very far away; later she tries to get a prescription filled for birth control pills, but is afraid because she knows the psychiatrist will check around and track her down through the pharmacies.

I tried to work on the dream but Ginny was strongly resistant. It seemed to interest me more than her; her resistance smothered her curiosity. I told her the dream reminded me of something we have often discussed—her feelings that only by being crazy can she possess my attention and concern. I asked, "Why would I tell you not to have children and not to move far away? Whose voice was it telling you that?" She says she doesn't know, it is almost like her parents' voice, but she knows that it's not her parents saying this now. They would like her to get married; so we came to the conclusion that the voice was her parents' voice speaking to her when she was a child, and that voice still continues alive in her. That was all. Another rich dream vein goes unmined.

Why hadn't she mentioned the cast on my leg? She said at first she hadn't noticed it was a cast, she thought it was just a piece of bandage. I asked her what it made her think of. She said it looked uncomfortable—I was sitting in unusual clothes and she could see the outline of my body more clearly—did I have on knit pants? She had a fantasy of my watching television with my pyjamas on. Underneath the pyjamas she saw something that looked like white underwear, which was a cast. Her thoughts were scattered, hard to follow. She never explicitly stated why she chose to ignore the cast. I can only assume that the cast, and the leg therein, brings her too close to the sexual strings between us.

She abruptly told me that Karl had said to her, "If you ever have a child, its first words will be 'I can't.'" (So my earlier intuition was correct: the word "impregnable" was not without significance; it cropped up in the dream, and when she talked about something missing in her life, she was thinking of the lack of children.) Karl's statement about her unborn child was cruel—cruel on more than one level. I asked why she hadn't said so to Karl; by not telling him, she was only proving what he had implied: that she can't do anything, can't even express her disapproval. Later on she said she liked my saying that sort of thing and that's what she wanted me to do. I accepted the invitation by pursuing the phantoms of marriage and children, forcing Ginny to face them with me. "What do you want from Karl? Do you want to get married? Do you want children? Why don't you ask him to marry you or at least find out what your status is? Are you going to be a common-law wife?" She said, "Oh, he would live with me for five years and 360 days and then leave just before the time expires." "Why do you put up with this? Either change the situation or stop complaining about it." She deftly cut my string of questions by saying in a comical way, "Listen to you with your sprained knee." And we both burst into laughter.

She said she really doesn't want to marry Karl because she still nourishes the fantasy of living alone in a cottage in the middle of a forest. I refused to be deflected and said that her fantasy was child-like and romantic and, besides, in her fantasy world she's never alone anyway; there is always some big person there looking out for her. Who is that big person? Why would he spend his life caring for her? Had he once been her father? Her father is not going to be present for her forever; one day he will be dead and she will have to continue living. This brought tears to her eyes and she murmured that she doesn't want to think that far ahead, but I assured her that this is one of the stark facts of life, which she must inevitably confront.

Earlier in the meeting, I had the feeling of her rebelling against me and rebuking me for being a crazy psychiatrist, who, unlike most psychiatrists, was getting her to look out rather than in. When I told her she looks in too much, she said she looked in with a superficial glance and wished I would stop criticizing her for being so introspective. All of this seemed like a healthy sign in that she's able to take some stand against me. One other thing that came up was that she noticed Madeline Greer's name on one of the other offices and said I should be careful not to say anything to Madeline because she knows her. Irony of ironies! Madeline, a colleague of mine, is the only person who has ever read any of Ginny's notes. It turns out that Madeline is now dating one of Ginny's friends. What to do? I am too mortified to tell Ginny and reluctant to discuss the matter with Madeline for fear of telling her more than she knows—I'm not sure she had connected the Ginny of the reports with the Ginny she met in San Francisco.

November 1

GINNY

WHEN I went into session, I had no particular problems or grievances and thought that everything was just going to be abstract. But I enjoyed the session and found it helpful, maybe because you talked more than usual.

Of course, it's only when we get to maudlin topics that I respond. Like when you said I'm going to have to live half my life without my parents. It's true I'm more dependent on them than most people my age because I still refer to myself in past contexts, not recognizing any change or growth. I mean I don't have a job that defines me, or another family. So I still feel like a free-lance *special* child.

When you did your little diatribe about my being special, I knew it was outrageous and you were half-putting me on, but it's true. That must be the way I see myself. And it's the special-ness that makes me reward myself with special fantasies of despair, solitude, a spinster spine that curls in upon itself. What I find most helpful in session is when I tell you something exact I've done and you show me alternative ways I could have reacted to the situation. This reinforces other modes of behavior. Like when I told you about Karl saying the first words a child of mine would ever say would be "I can't" and my only reaction was hurt, and then fear, and a need to sidle up to him and see if he still liked me. When I behave that skunky way, I have to fantasize that the real me isn't what's there every day, and that when I have no one to sidle up to and please and need, I'll find real punishment and real salvation. This stops me from trying to change my behavior everyday and right now. It's when I can experiment with everyday life and change my old patterns that I feel I've succeeded and grown. I don't really want to go into exile and self-torture. I like Karl and my surroundings and need all that.

November 9

DR. YALOM

A LACKLUSTER HOUR, rather plodding, with no real peaks of interest. Ginny began by saying that she had had a bad time last night for a stupid reason; it started when Karl said he wasn't feeling well because he is concerned about his future and his career. This occurred just before they went to bed. Once in bed, she started having fantasies of his leaving her and became upset at the thought of being all alone. This incident set the tone of the rest of the meeting since my associations were immediately that she should have found out what was troubling Karl and then tried to do something to help him. When I implied as much, she responded by asking "What could I have done? What would your wife have done?" I groaned, "Oh, no!" And then she turned it into a joke by saying, "What would Mrs. Nixon have said to President Nixon?" I guess I never went back to her question, in one way because I didn't think it would help Ginny to know what my wife would have said, but also because Ginny was asking for some personal information which I balked at giving. At any rate, it soon took us to the fact that she and Karl don't talk personally about anything. It would never dawn upon Ginny to help Karl explore his feelings about his future, and I'm sure this is, in part, why she can't obtain any clarity from him about their future together. There are strong rules in their relationship which prevent serious personal talk of any nature from occurring, although they talk about ideas quite splendidly for hours on end. I felt her straining for instruction as to how she should break this pattern with Karl. I asked her what she wants to know from him, which led her to what I think is the crucial question: What does their relationship mean to Karl? How long and how deeply is he going to commit himself to it?

She then talked about a literary party where she acted like a ten-year-old girl in the presence of some older people; she froze up because she felt she had no essence. If Karl hadn't been there, if other people hadn't been there, she would simply have curled up and become nothing because all she felt she could do was bounce off

115

other people's ideas. I shared with her my belief that it's really quite the contrary, that she has an extremely powerful essence which one always senses and recognizes. When she hears the "adults" talk, she can't carry on a conversation with them, but is perfectly able to sit back and satirize it in her mind. Her conduct didn't seem so very unreasonable to me; why does she have to be the same as everyone else socially? She then trapped me very deftly by retorting that if that's the way she is, why am I expecting her to change in her relationship with Karl? I squirmed out of that one by arguing that people can be different socially, but when they relate closely to one another, they generally have to talk about intimate matters, unless they are so busy surviving or working together that they are personal without talking about it. She and Karl spend so much time talking with others about their inmost feelings and exploring them in their writing, it seems inconceivable to me that they can continue to be with one another unless, at some level, they communicate more personally.

Ginny said that the last small change in her life occurred when I forced her to talk to Karl about the gasoline money—it was a painful, but somehow an extremely important shift in their relationship. She wishes I would force her to do something like that again.

There was a time today when I felt that Ginny had practically nothing more to say to me, indicating that maybe she's better, maybe she will be discontinuing therapy before long. Certainly, there are problem areas, but all and all her life is beginning to assume a more satisfying pattern.

November 9

GINNY

I BROUGHT UP the topics of conversation—my inability to talk with Karl about serious things, for example. This is part of my one-dimensional nature, and I think the way I behave with him is the way I do with you. So to know how Karl feels—how do you feel? (I should have asked) and how long will you both last? Of course I have more fear with Karl, since more of my vital time and organs and feelings are involved.

When you asked if I had learned anything from the group, that took me by surprise. None of my experiences are stepping stones or progressions. I used the group for the temporary companionship but anyway we didn't ask too many questions in the group that got truly answered, and any questions asked toward me, I never answered too well. I break down on a rational line, am more a vicious circle in the shape of a grin. We had two silences yesterday but they were blank silences—you ask what's happening and I say nothing.

I was glad Madeline had spoken to you and I imagined (not asking you) she said I was sweet. But see, I confuse being serious with confession. When I met her at the party I was acting like a paralyzed ingenue (my mother said that you can do your "nothing act" at a party but don't stand in one place so people become aware of it). So after Karl brought you up at the party and Madeline was encouraging, I told her I had been going to you for three years; that this year I was writing for you. Now I didn't have to or want to say that, but when I can't think of anything to say, I just tell anything pertinent to the other person.

What you said yesterday about having to speak up was right but it had no emotional impact, got no further than a magazine article. You and I just didn't get through to me. I didn't feel too badly.

Walking to the station I felt optimistic, imagining I had already spoken to Karl and everything was fine. Then in my fantasy animation you had to go on a business trip and postponed next session, and so I called you up and said how good everything was.

See how my mind dawdles or shortcuts all serious work and problems.

Even though I'm so on the outside, when we talked about my "presence," I liked it. But I know I need a special cadre around me to feel natural, to have any presence. I can't force myself to talk even when I'm making other people uncomfortable by my silence. I can't give. They have to give to me. I know this isn't important but still I feel spoiled that I can't give the minimum in ordinary situations.

November 16

DR. YALOM

A RATHER single-minded interview today and one which was quite uncomfortable for me. I felt like a cheerleader or a second in a boxing corner egging Ginny on. Essentially, she came in to say that she hadn't done what I had suggested last week—she hadn't been able to bring up the question of marriage to Karl—and ironically enough an opportunity to do so had fortuitously been dropped in her lap. One of her friends had cornered Karl and Ginny at a party and asked, half comically, "When are you two going to get married?" Karl immediately replied that he's not interested in marriage, that he doesn't call what Ginny and he have a "marriage." Ginny said the opportunity to talk to him about it that night was lost when she impulsively invited everyone over to their house to watch a movie on T.V. until 4 a.m. Karl was so angry at her for doing this that the evening ended with her having to apologize to him to assuage his anger rather than vice-versa.

A couple of other troubling incidents arose; for example, the other night Karl began to chew her out for having made a mistake in preparing some part of the dinner, and started haranguing her about her many weaknesses. She meekly agreed with everything he said and practically thanked him for telling her. I tried to go over alternative things she could have said, wondering mainly how it came about that their relationship was so defined that he had the right to criticize her without her having the reciprocal prerogative. She said, well, she could start telling him some of the things he did wrong, but it was pointless because the fact is that he was absolutely right in his criticism. I had to keep repeating over and over again: it isn't whether he was right or not, but how did the relationship get defined in that manner? I did some role playing with her, repeating what Karl had said and asking her to respond in a different way. She then began to make excuses, saying that she was just trying to make him a gourmet dinner, or would he rather have hamburgers, which she could make without a single mistake? I told her she was being very indirect; couldn't she say anything more personal? In the safety of my office she role-played. She told Karl that he had hurt her; why did he have to cut her down just before they went to bed?

Then she slipped out of that uncomfortable scene with the comical observation that she felt as if I were putting her through a Samurai school, teaching her how to have her feet planted in the right place, and how to hold the sword.

She told me of another incident in which she had blurted out "I love you" to Karl during the week and Karl had made no answer, and I wondered why she didn't feel she had the right to inquire into his silence. She insisted she knows the answer already—that he does not love her and is not interested in marrying her. Then I made two observations. The first was, if that were true, is she interested in remaining with Karl? Is this "loveless" relationship all that she wants in life? Secondly, I told her I have absolutely no faith in her ability to collect data. As an example, I reminded her that she had for a long time been unable to ask me to switch the hour of our meeting because she thought it would upset me and when she finally screwed up her courage enough to ask, she found out that she had been completely wrong in her perceptions—the same may very well be true of Karl. She's overlooking many things, such as the fact that he has spent a good portion of his adult life with her. And so we went on with my pushing her and pushing her and pushing her to "say something personal" to Karl. I have some fears about how this will go, and maybe I'm asking her to do something she can't do, and maybe this relationship with Karl is better than none at all. I guess in the background of my thoughts is the memory of Madeline's telling me how hostile a person she thought Karl was when she met him. Maybe I'm overly protective of Ginny but it does seem that Karl's crapping all over her and I do somehow want to rescue her from this guy or at least help her alter the relationship so that it will be more livable for her.

November 16

GINNY

PERHAPS it's a better sign that I don't remember too much about what happened yesterday. Sitting waiting for you I saw a tear-stained girl leave her therapist and I felt those were the good old days, my past, "wet tissues, big issues."

Anyway by the time we started I had filled myself with anxiety, sure I had nothing to talk about, sure I had to go to the bathroom. And felt that all I could do is tell you things that were over, not meant for change. And then as we started talking, I knew I would cry, especially when talking of that evening with Bud questioning us about marriage. And I kept talking, but concentrating, gloating, filled with my own trembling. And I kept this up a long time until I finally put the spark out with my own tears. See, I'm not as interested in the discussions as I am in the feelings they elicit. The tears are much easier to have than the intelligence behind them.

And we came back to our old subject "Why can't I talk up?" By now you were playing Karl's part, but I never really played mine. (Although I remember now that's what I keep asking you, to give me a chance to pretend what I would do.) I know it's a safe situation inside the office but I don't push myself. At least you make me feel that I will never be kicked or thrown out. So like when you say, "You'll never stand up for yourself unless you can see that you yourself can get out of the situation, that you have some say," I knew that was important, that I should remember and think about it, but I filed it away under "another day."

Somehow I felt like I had taken several steps closer to a starting line from where we could begin. Even though I could have begun that very day, I didn't. I knew I was just talking on after a certain point had been reached. As usual I rationed my reactions and sensations. I was unable to concentrate. Perhaps I should have told you the exact moment I strayed and we could have talked about that. But instead I watched you trying to incite me, trying to get me to move. But I already felt cozy and soggy as if I had just been lowered into a crib.

When I kept saying "I feel dead," I felt dead. All that was annoying you and I felt ashamed how often it slipped out as an excuse. And I know if I would stop thinking I were dead, I would be more open to feelings underneath. Which I definitely think I had at last week's session.

You seemed very impatient with some of my "apologies for the past," as you called them.

November 23

DR. YALOM

A TERRIBLE SESSION with Ginny today but to make it worse it comes right on the heels of an equally bad session with another patient. My other patient was very hostile, resistive, silent and distrustful of me, and I kept trying to provoke her into some form of activity.

With Ginny there was an absolute dearth of anything to grab hold of or work on. I gradually was overcome by a seeping feeling of futility of ever helping Ginny change; she doesn't want to make any changes in herself. At the end of the hour I felt I was facing an absolutely smooth stone cliff with only the tiniest chink in it for a foothold and that chink was my saying once more to Ginny that she is unhappy because she doesn't know whether Karl is ever going to marry her and why doesn't she ask him? That seemed to be the only possible therapeutic ledge, and it had already been worn very thin.

She came in. The first sentence was that she had been feeling great until she walked into this office. Then she stated that she has been typing up her story and sending it around to magazines. It was obvious that she was ashamed of not having followed my prescription of talking to Karl personally. To prevent me from scolding her she offered me a reward in the form of her story. Naturally I could have pointed this out to her, but so what? Much of the rest of the hour was spent with Ginny lamenting the fact that she wasn't "serious," that she shouldn't talk at all because she is just babbling, without really working on anything. She and I were so impersonal and distant through all this that I finally invited her to ask me something directly. She finally said, "How long will you continue to see me, continue to let me come and babble and say I'm feeling fine?" I tried to answer her openly and honestly by replying that I would see this through with her and that I didn't take very seriously her assertions that all was well when there are such obvious major areas of dissatisfaction in her life. She seemed rather gleeful at that news, just like a small child. Later on she said that she was disgusted with herself, she wasn't "leveling" with me, she felt like a phony, even the ends of her smiles felt phony. I couldn't do anything at all to help her. I just repeated over and over the question: "Do you want to change?" Perhaps the status quo is too comfortable. I feel as though all responsibility for change is being placed in my lap. She even wants me to set her goals for her. I must have said the same thing in four or five different ways, but all to no avail. Today I had for the first time the thought that I've left therapy too open-ended. Maybe I should just set a termination date, four months, six months. It would probably speed up our work. I wonder sometimes whether she wants me to do this. Perhaps she was asking for it today.

November 23

GINNY

BEFORE I went in I was afraid there was nothing to talk about, but then I thought like magic it would work itself out. It would have, if I hadn't been so talkative and rigid. I was apologizing from the word go. I couldn't be spontaneous and change a bad situation or think my way out of it. Maybe what I did in session is what I'm doing here—just talking about myself in a selfish way. It was one of the most uncomfortable times.

When I said that I wanted you to correct me and give me goals, I didn't mean household chores to fill my week—that would be too immediate and petty; but I wanted things to do while in the office. Everything that happens comes from the impetus to talk to you about what you think is important. You are the master of ceremonies. So I blame you for our constant picking away at the same old scabs, the same old crucial obviousness—does he love or even like me, will Karl leave me? It's like going over the same charade sentence in the same way.

I was a vacuum inside yesterday. My life has settled like tumbleweed against a boundary fence and I am just catching my breath, until the next wind and upheaval. Now sitting here at home without your comfort, I can think of lots of things to say.

About the boredom and pressure of this existence. How Karl, before he gets into bed at night, will sometimes scale the walls with his eyes, scan our home and say, "I hate this place. I hate it." And I can't believe he is not really scanning me, using the house as a scapegoat to speak to me. That doesn't leave me with a feeling of love and abandon, and even when I can reach out and tell him in a satiric way how that statement is just not love-inducing before bed, and is kind of cruel, I am left with a great feeling of uneasiness and dissatisfaction that he uses sentences like that, knows their impact, and is just not sensitive or caring about us. And then I can think that he's going through really bad times himself, and is lashing out. Or maybe I had no problems to solve yesterday. I felt like I was wasting both our times.

When you asked about goals I realized how outside any self I feel. I gave civic answers. I might as well have been talking to a high school guidance counselor.

I didn't bother to listen to you when I was sort of interested in your opinions, like when we were talking about my savings account. I use my savings account like my talent. I let it sit there collecting interest, afraid to spend it except minimally and spontaneously, while waiting for that emergency when I will need my soul and money. Once again putting off. Saving myself for the crisis or fatality.

I felt doubly bad thinking of the write-up afterwards. There's so little to work with when what we're talking about is things not done, rather than things done and gone wrong. But I felt a little angry that the whole session got off on the wrong feet because I hadn't talked to Karl. I guess I set it up that way by acting childishly and telling you about my writing as something to please you. But why couldn't you change it?

You used to be able to relax me and try different ways when things weren't working. The session felt like an interview where I was applying for a job I didn't want.

A session like that is always contagious and half-way through I knew I would punish myself afterwards, which I did. And that's what depresses me—that I can't stop this, that I can't ask you to help me, that I let me go on.

I should get angry when you keep baiting me with the status

quo by saying maybe I'm happy. I guess I'm supposed to leap up at that point and say, "no no, it's rotten." But I don't and that's supposed to mean nothing's wrong. You yourself said it isn't a successful status quo but that maybe I don't mind.

Well, I don't really want to give up my life with Karl, though you and my own words push me toward it. I never tell you of the good times since they come easily, naturally and are gone. And they are bordered on every side by our silence, our inability to really say we need and love each other. . . .

I was justy putty in that chair trying to feign emotions and shape.

November 30

DR. YALOM

A VERY SAD little hour. Things seem to grow more and more bleak. I feel discouraged, impotent, puzzled about which way to turn. Every once in awhile there is a brief ray of hope which then doesn't carry me very far. I sometimes feel as though we share an illusion; both of us know it's all hopeless but we never dare speak the word.

She started off by saying that a few days after the last session one of her best friends complained that she, Ginny, never really reveals anything about herself. Her friend has no way of knowing what Ginny is thinking or feeling. Since then Ginny's been trying to be more open, but feels coerced, even though her friend did not present it as an ultimatum. Obviously this parallels what I have been saying to her these many months. There's a bit of hopefulness in it since, as she pointed out later in the hour, this at least gives her someone else besides me with whom she can try to be different.

Then she went on to tell me how miserable she's been since the last session, which was so terrible for both of us. Immediately thereafter she experienced a devastating sense of finality, as if she had received a score marked with indelible ink on her forehead and she could never change it. "Why not say to yourself, 'So what? The hour was a bummer! What's final about that?'"

Something interesting, though, to whet my appetite for intellectual stimulation. Since the last hour she has been absolutely obsessed with fantasies, most of which are on the general theme of her life in the future. She is thirty, perhaps thirty-five years old, living alone, miserable, unhappy, working at some menial job, like in a department store. Occasionally people see her, maybe I or her parents see her, and then the fantasy is terminated by her going into a long weeping spell in which she feels great self-pity. I kept asking myself as she describes this to me, what purpose is this fantasy serving? The fantasy must be a wish. What would the wish be? My guess is that in being unhappy, she would make me and her parents and Karl unhappy. There's clearly a great deal of hostility in this fantasy. I told her about a scene in one of Beckett's plays where the protagonist wishes his parents are in heaven, but also hopes they are able to see him suffering down in hell. None of the interpretations about hostility made any impact upon her. When I pressed them a little harder in the interview, she admitted to having felt that perhaps I should have done something different last time, that I should have used some relaxation techniques, or maybe she should be in behavioral therapy. That almost verged on criticism. I remarked on it, but in so doing, extinguished it.

We ended up the session on the familiar theme of her inability to speak personally to Karl. What's happening now is that Karl is unable to find a job. He applies for one after the other, is always turned down and is sinking deeper into depression. She does pride herself on the fact that once this week when he was lying on the bed, she asked him what was the matter. He said that he was just down, but that it was something about him and not about Ginny. I wondered why, during all this period, she hasn't given him more opportunity to talk about the pain he is obviously feeling. To me it is very much like a child whose father is out of a job and not allowed to be privy to such adult matters. She said that this is indeed the way she feels. Any kind of change just devastates her. She recalls that when she was five years old and her father left a job at Sears, she went into hysterics at the news. Is she simply unable to face the idea of some sort of change in her relationship with Karl? She knows that they are hurtling toward a crisis. Karl obviously can't continue out of work, and if he doesn't find a job soon, something will happen, he may leave town or leave her. But she dare not ask.

She's also gotten a full-time Christmas job for the next three weeks and will probably not meet with me during this period. I didn't have any strong feelings about this, one way or the other. I'm a little sad not to see her, but also I feel so discouraged and pessimistic right now that I welcome the reprieve.

She was making some effort to be a little closer by looking at me very directly and saying that at least she could do that, make that much contact with me.

January 18

DR. YALOM

I HAVEN'T SEEN Ginny for a month. She has been working at a book store over the Christmas holidays. Within a very few minutes we are back into the same familiar dreary mire. To be with Ginny is a unique dramatic experience. It's as though she brings her own gray stage setting and deftly arranges it in the first moments of the hour. Very soon I am caught up in the drama. I experience the world as she does: a strange, uncanny, circular despondency. I begin to share her hopelessness. In today's session it took the form of, "I can never be happy with Karl because I can't have an orgasm any more and I can't have an orgasm because these voices keep ridiculing me when I try to have an orgasm." The "voices" are only the shrieks of her own self-hatred, and the more she fails, at orgasm and all else, the more persistent and the louder the shrieks become. And so the snake devours its tail. And there's no way out. And my head begins to swim after ten or fifteen minutes. And I feel helpless and irritable.

I tell her that she possibly never will have an orgasm during intercourse, that fifty percent of the women in the world probably don't have orgasms, that she's got the whole goddamn thing focused around whether or not she finds the magic orgasm. She has a ready argument for this, presented, of course, obsequiously: it's the women from the last generation who don't have orgasms and everything she reads in the newspapers now demonstrates that women are having more orgasms. It sounds almost comical, but in a sense she's right. I have maneuvered myself into an untenable position. What I wanted to emphasize are the positive aspects of her life: she's working and earning money, her relationship to Karl has blossomed, he has become extremely affectionate and caring, but she says she can't imagine marrying him because she can't have an orgasm with him. That blows my mind. She supports her position by citing the number of divorces on the grounds of "incompatibility." I want to point out that incompatibility is not necessarily a missing orgasm, but what's the use, this is getting us nowhere.

Last night she had a sudden weeping spell for which she could find no explanation. Today she has a headache. Last week when she called me she was glad I couldn't give her an appointment until this week. Obviously she's got mixed feelings about coming back to see me, but we couldn't pursue them very far.

Then she described a recurring fantasy concerning Karl and her girlfriend; she wishes her girlfriend would invite her over to the house but tell her not to bring Karl. She imagines how upset she would be at her friend and the angry things she would say to her. Then she fantasized being at home alone in the evenings feeling sorry for herself, while Karl was at the poolhall. (The only reason for such fantasies is that aggression committed against her would permit her to feel justified in aggressing back, if only in a fantasy.) I gave her a simplistic interpretation that all her behavior is explicable in terms of her unexpressed anger. I told her that her fantasies, her inability to take care of herself in any form, her overtimidity, her respectfulness with me, her refusal ever to hurt anyone, her refusal to find out from Karl what he intends for the future—all stem from her stifled anger. She responded by saying that this has been a wonderfully long interview. I pointed out that of all the things she could have chosen to say to me, she picked a compliment. Well, this made some sense to her and Ginny was terribly interested, as was I. However, we both realized that it's nothing new and in fact we have talked about her unexpressed anger countless times, more times than I care to remember. It really makes me think again of the word "cyclotherapy." Ginny seems to feel, however, that her anger may be getting a little closer to the surface, that the smoldering irritation is a bit more real to her than it has been in the past. I don't know if this really is the case or if Ginny was offering up her anger to placate my general sense of discouragement.

January 18

GINNY

I WAS NOT sarcastic within myself during the session. I concentrated on what I was saying or thinking and this gave me energy. So it didn't seem to drag ever. I covered so much— the vacation, my work, the new shoes, bedtime, Eve. Then Dr. Yalom finally tied them all up together (I am consciously going to call you Dr. Yalom from here on. Calling you "you" makes it seem like you're just sitting across from me and so I strive to please you and delight you and if I do criticize you, it's with a smirk on my face. But your real name might put a distance there and I'll stop performing.). I realize I try to compliment Dr. Yalom, as at the end when I said, "this session has been wonderfully long," and Dr. Yalom reared up. It hadn't dawned on me but I realize now I skirted away from what he was putting before me to respond as though everything were over and the bow was tied.

At the session anger was brought up again. Thinking about anger I can tie it in even more strongly and help understand my berserk, nervous childish behavior at work. I always asked one too many questions and put myself in a position to gently infuriate anyone. I couldn't just have a normal interchange, no, I had to go several beats further. I was like a shadow who leaves a stupid grinning body in the way of danger. A punching bag of vapor.

I always knew I was doing wrong, putting my foot in it, yet I seemed helpless to stop myself. I probably enjoy feeling this self-spite.

In sessions I do it too, but some of it must be ingenuous to you, since it doesn't seem to anger you outright. For instance, telling you I like coming for therapy because I've found a place that makes good black and white sodas and a discount drug store. Dr. Yalom doesn't defend himself, his time against my yapping. I bare myself, I expose myself to see how small I can become. I have no internal plan, no *self*-preservation, or the self I'm trying to preserve is already a fossil. I was always scared to step out of line at work and did exactly what was prescribed —taking no responsibility for any self-motivation. In sessions too I probably wait for you to start the ball rolling. In fact I do.

Immediately after session I thought of a picture of myself that I would like to give you, a symbolic pose, so I guess at the very end I was thinking to please you, and ingratiate myself with you once again because it's a pretty picture.

I'm glad I talked again about the mess of consciousness, the tangled scrambling voices that bombard me when I'm making love, and I hope he realized as I did when I tried to explain that it is no longer the orgasm or lack of it that is such a big issue but the confusion and hatred that I reap on myself, that fill me up. Even when I enjoy myself and feel great pleasure as afterwards when I usually get excited again with Karl still in me, it's like a clandestine pleasure—one I'm not sure Karl would approve of or understand, he'd wonder why I couldn't come with him, why I dawdled so. He'd think it is only second best, which it is, a situation that somehow I've confined myself to. Especially since it used to be uncomplicated.

When I talked about the word "incompatible" I think Dr. Yalom thought I was pulling his leg, which I wasn't. I believed what I said, he doesn't realize how technically childish I am or stay or try to be. He'll never convince me though that *that* part of life—sex—isn't one of the most important. And I can't get by by blotting it out, and concentrating on the kitchen table. While Karl is wrong in so many of his schoolmasterish habits, in bed he is able most times to be free and forgetting, if not forgiving. Then it doesn't matter how many dinners and books and words I serve up to Karl, if I can't give him myself purely, and completely, without feeling like I'm mimicking a woman.

I was with Dr. Yalom all the way, until the time when he changed the topic from sex to my general relationship. Then that seemed too big and rangy a topic to cope with and I couldn't think about it. But I will try this week. I'll rehearse, if need be, since he'll bring it up again and again. I guess I don't leave Dr. Yalom much leeway with my censored topics. I refuse to talk about any blame my parents might have. Whenever he baits me or I bait myself and say "the ugly women were after me making sarcastic remarks," he says, "Who are these ugly women? Have you ever known them?" and the issue gets fuzzy and we move on. We are both being transparent. Never give a psychiatrist an even break.

He is always talking about assertiveness toward others, but I feel safer thinking of assertiveness within myself. To control my own thoughts. (That way no one will get attacked but my innards.) I know Dr. Yalom disapproves when I express my goal to control my thoughts and integrate them and at the same time still smoke grass. (I don't deny him his sherry.) When I smoke grass, the dry thoughts and sentences I have, actually get a taste and feel. The thoughts released are already there and are just loosened up and animated, allowed to scramble around and become fascinating and real. They're simmering ingredients already in the stew, so why ignore them?

Are you just looking at a phenomenon that will not change, or do you think I can change? I know you're answering yes, "but in small ways." And I am coming to see that that would be fine, because it's the small things that cancel my good feelings and make me so frustrated till I could die.

Addition to January 18

I told you I would show you the kind of thing I write when I get in my frustrated, bleak mood. Here is something I wrote recently.

I took a walk to a street that was safe behind garages, a kind of weedy mews. No traffic bulldozes the silence. The only noises are the close birds and the faraway mindless fog horns. The road slopes up. It has been paved privately and raspberry bushes disguise it. Also green and yellow grass, nephews to weeds hide in it. And I, too, hide. I came for a retreat. From up here the part of the city by the bay looks like shells shallowly covered by tide, as the fog drowns all the rough edges of downtown and leaves a standing white tower like some child's sand toy. Till night crashes in.

A few days before my period I always get mad. Maybe it's the new difference between working and not working. (I'm unemployed now.) My body is swift and tireless but in three rooms begins to sag and putter. I have at least two tennis sets in me today but no partner and the walks, this walk, is limited by lack of purpose. Karl is an enigma. I don't know if it's my bad mood constructing him into worse things or his own stinginess shining through. He can spend fifteen dollars on cards and when I ask to go out to dinner, not paid for, just accompanied, his face turns a sickly negative. Then I get angry at myself, it's my fault to bring up dinner when he's unemployed. My fierce concentration on leisure escapes. This lopsided eagerness to fill my life with pastimes, hinging on other people. And always a draught.

Then seeing Larry again (an old lover) who gave me an incomplete scenario to be loved and beautiful again. I stood stiffly by him giving him my smile, allowing myself only baby steps and an instant replay afterwards. Anger toward other people, I let it beat in me and grow like sexual excitement. And resentment and hate. That's how I thrash myself to sleep. Saying half syllables to God, wishing He would clean my mind and soul of so many indictments and images. My behavior is a reminiscent dream of the worst scenes.

This lack of initiative and personal belief makes me feel most a victim when I am being treated nicely, because I think "How kind of you, how merciful, but for this, this movie or dinner or call or dress, and I would be coiled in on myself ready to spring and bite hard."

But I fence these overripe feelings off. I make a Greek potato-tomato skillet, and so playing the little Miss, I find salvation and a mercy of vitamins.

January 25

DR. YALOM

A CURIOUSLY playful, informal hour with Ginny. It's especially puzzling to me why that was so since I was exceedingly upset before the session. Three hours before Ginny came in I had an extremely disturbing session with another patient, which finally ended in my doing the one thing I try never to do—acting irresponsibly, maybe even destructively, by completely losing my temper. The patient ran out of the office. Afterwards I felt guilty because this patient has been depressed and sleepless, and an additional disturbance is the last thing she needs. Of course I can rationalize it in a lot of different ways: my getting angry might be helpful to her, her contempt and anger would have taxed the patience of St. Francis, a therapist is only human. No matter, after she left I was shaken and seriously concerned she might do something drastic, possibly even attempt suicide.

During the two hours between her session and Ginny's I had a meeting with the psychiatric residents, which gave me little time to reflect upon the incident, so that coming to see Ginny, I began to dwell upon it and initially was deeply distracted. However, it was very comforting to see Ginny, and I managed to forget Ann, the other patient. I guess Ginny is so unlike Ann, so nonthreatening, so very grateful for any little thing I give her, that it made me feel comfortable to be with her. I live the drama of "Rosencrantz and Guildenstern"; there's another play offstage, other actors in the wings. I could be writing a scenario starring Ann, with only a bit part for Ginny. That's the ultimate and terrible secret of the psychotherapist—the dramas on the other stage.

I'm writing this the next day and it's hard for me to get the sequence of events clear in my mind. What I remember most, as I look back on the hour, was that I felt Ginny to be more adult, less grinning, more buxom, more attractive. What's more I told her all these things. I encouraged her to ask me some questions, as if that would be a more grown-up way of our being together. She started off the interview very quickly by asking me what was wrong. I denied there was anything wrong, but later on I told her that I had been upset by another patient. Her response was a peculiar one. It was almost as if she were sad because she couldn't imagine my getting angry with *her* and I told her that was true. Then she went on to talk about the fantasies she's had all week, which were just like the fantasies of the week before—setting up situations in which she could be angry with people. I do think our insights into her hidden anger have been useful because we now have a clearer grasp of what this deluge of fantasies means.

She is very much aware of feeling and acting like a little girl and of her constant grinning. Today she really stopped grinning for almost the entire hour, and I felt decidedly different about her. She has gained a lot of weight, she said, and naturally turned that into something destructive with the irrational conviction that she's going to be the same weight as her mother and resents the thought that she may have her mother's unfavorable traits without any of the favorable ones. This is a typical example of Ginny's magical thinking. I responded only by letting her know how irrational I thought that was, and how she turns any factor into something negative for herself. I insisted that she actually looked much better. I almost found myself being somewhat seductive to her. It's interesting to note that when she left my office, a friend who came in to chat for a moment commented on the "attractive girl" who had just walked out.

Another question she asked was whether or not I would please pretend to be twenty years younger. I told her I could not do that without a great deal of embarrassment. She then asked me quasi-seriously to plan out her week for her and tell her exactly what she should do. I responded in kind and gave her several suggestions: talk openly with Karl, write two hours a day, stop grinning. Another subject she brought up entailed what I considered a bizarre way of looking at her relationship with Karl. Karl is very depressed, out of a job, and Ginny has a feeling that he will blame her for this, as if she has "pulled him down." To my mind, it is much more likely that he will see her from exactly the opposite viewpoint, i.e., now that everything else has fallen down about him, she's the only thing he has. In fact, there's some evidence for this position, since he has recently been much more affectionate with her. At the end of the hour she asked about reading my latest write-ups and I promised that I'd get them together for next week. A refreshing, loose, free time with Ginny.

January 25

GINNY

I THINK I wasn't looking forward to therapy as I had nothing definite on my mind and didn't know what I could say. Before the session, as I told you, I felt tranced, as if I could sit staring for hours. But after only ten minutes the session began.

Dr. Yalom acted strangely, sitting low in his chair and smiling, with his hand covering his mouth in my pauses. Later he said he was feeling nervous and told me why, which I found interesting. I pictured the scene briefly, some girl being sarcastic to him time after time and him finally getting angry. I wondered why something like that hadn't happened between us—what with my slow progress in circles. And God I am sarcastic, not toward him but myself. He said it would be hard to find my anger (which sounds like a great phrase). In other words he couldn't be angry with me unless I, like the girl, had been ceaselessly angry at him. The thought was very exciting. Then I realized how limited our scenario was as a result of me and the therapy— just up on my little perch where I can't be touched except by certain gentle emotions, innuendos and whimsy. Maybe that's why there's such a loud bitch in me, because I have to supply all the bad things to myself, all the real life hard knocks feed-back. I'm not exposed to a tenth of the spectrum of emotions that other people are. I envy emotions and girls who run out or are bodily thrown out of psychiatrists' offices.

I kept talking on and on, had no idea how it was coming across, so believed the worst. I wasn't plumbing any new feelings. But Dr. Yalom sat so quietly, yet with a lot of expressions on his face, that I thought he must be getting dizzy with my droning and searching for a topic. When I asked him what he was thinking, he said I seemed better. He could respond more to me this way than at other times. If he had said I was awful and talking nonsense, I could gladly have believed that too. I had no judgment. When I asked why I seemed better, I had no inkling up my sleeve. He said I seemed better because "you are more serious. You're acting ten years older, you're more buxom." I had just told him about my ten more pounds of weight since last session. He said a sentence I wish I could quote but I've already imagined it wrong, something like "you look better, more buxom, more womanly and you're not grinning."

I didn't allow myself any sensual response or afterthought until later. We had been talking about the angry girl and how she got his angry response. And I said, at least that way she gets responses, and he said, yes but I don't have to respond to you that way. There are other ways. (pause) And one part of me was touched and pleased and excited by the great implications and compliment. And another was sarcastic and funny, not uttering anything on the audible level, but so used to its own jokes, not having to say "Oh ya buddy. That's what they all say." Later all this had a good effect, somehow I did feel better, more serious, whole and joyful. Trekking back through the woods passing Stanford's grave, I was different from the genius in- genue I usually am. I was a womanly type, eating hors d'oeuvres and drinking from a crystal glass in one hand and Dr. Yalom and his wife and some friends (in the other hand)? and talk- ing and mature. But the world seemed clearer, I was concentrating, I was alive. Standard time is wearing off so it really was lighter at 5:15. The world was light. When I got home I was full of fun and joy and when Karl touched my paunch and I came up with some quip, he said "What did your shrink say to you today?" (I was prancing around by then) I said he had told me how womanly I was. "So that's the kind of things he says," said Karl with just as much fun.

P.S. Key words in session—good tact, good timing. There will always be conflict between the ideals of openness, love, gut reaction, the great universal hard things (as I imagine and dream of them from afar) and obtainable therapy goals (maybe the others are the realm of religion) but I believe in the first, maybe as a shield against having to work on the small things, the assign- able things, and as a way against admitting any success. And Dr. Yalom is always trying to show me that all people are hidden. Okay, maybe they are. But not all are afraid. I'm afraid with my hiding. Dr. Yalom is trying to make me feel comfortable with my bum rap.

February 1

DR. YALOM

A DIFFERENT KIND of session from last week. No playful seductive underpinnings to the interview but we were quite relaxed and going about our business in an adult way. She came in and told me (surprise of surprises) that she'd had a good week. No, on second thought she started off the interview in a discouraged tone. The first thing she said was that she had tried talking to Karl and it had failed. As she went on to describe the incident, it seems that she had indeed tried to talk personally to Karl but in a negative, critical fashion, and it had gone very badly. She was reading one of his short stories and commented that he speaks in an authoritarian way just like the characters in that story. He responded defensively, asked for some concrete examples, and ended up saying he was really too shaky for her to upset him like this. She concluded, therefore, that if he's too upset to talk about this, he'd be too upset to talk about even more important matters. However, everything else that she had to say about the week was generally encouraging. She took a trip to Yosemite with another couple and had a marvelous weekend. Karl hadn't gone because he wanted to do some writing. When she came home he told her how empty his life had been without her. It's quite clear to me, and to Ginny as well, how abruptly their relationship has switched. She is no longer in a position of great fear that he'll suddenly announce he is leaving her; the shoe is on the other foot, it's apparent that she's in the ascendant position and that he needs her at least as much as she needs him.

She then went on to say that the only thing that's really standing in her way now is the dread of night and of sex. I at first tried a rational approach, pointing out to her that that's really a small percentage of her life, a few minutes, at most an hour or two. She took an unusually brave stand against me, dug in her heels and retorted that that's a very misguided opinion on my part and all the popular magazines disagree with me. She pulled me up smartly. Well, then I proceeded to investigate with a good deal more seriousness (and I am taking Ginny more seriously) the whole issue of what's been happening in bed with Karl. We've gone over it many times, but this time I understood more clearly. Her night sexual terrors did not arise with her previous boyfriend because he would masturbate her. With Karl, in the beginning, things were good sexually, very natural. She didn't have to ask him to masturbate her. Then she started to tense up, to clutch and the vicious circle was drawn: tension blocked her spontaneity, she dreaded and berated herself for her lack of spontaneity, and more tension was generated. With Karl the primary problem is that she continues to be afraid to ask Karl to help her, she somehow thinks that he would object to doing certain things, would consider it kind of a defeat or a cheap way out. She explained the difference in the two men by saying that the first boyfriend was Jewish and that Jewish boys are more sensitive and conflicted about sex and anxious to please the girl because of their own particular conflicts with their Jewish mothers. What could I say to that streak of wisdom? She plunged me into thought about my own mother.

I surfaced and pressed her to investigate her fears; just what is she afraid of? It's clear that Karl will do nothing to harm her; what really stops her from approaching him? She described what usually happens at night. They go to bed holding each others' hands, each of them lying there, and she is afraid to say anything to him. If she said what she wanted, it would be to ask Karl to call her by name or to look at her or to hold her. I tried to persuade her to make some move toward him, to put her arm around him, or kiss him or tell him that she feels frightened and would like him to hold her. It is exactly this type of gesture which she finds most frightening. Then she blurted out, semi-jokingly, that she wasn't going to try anything like this when I was going to be out of town for two weeks. I had forgotten I was to be away. From everything Ginny said, I got the feeling that she feared this was her final step in therapy. What would happen to us, I asked, if she were able to talk intimately with Karl? What would she and I have to talk about? I said it half in jest and half seriously because I think it is crucially pertinent. She would rather stay in therapy than get well and give me up. However, she replied in a rather interesting fashion. She mused that she'd be something like her friend Eve. If she ever got past this, she'd have to begin seriously to consider her position outside, she'd have to beat her fists against the world, to find a career, to look for her place in life. I was stunned by her response because it means that Ginny is beginning to come close to thinking seriously about these issues. I don't think I've ever felt so strongly in all the time I've seen her that she has indeed changed. Suddenly she's begun to move very quickly.

And all this follows last week's "buxom" session. An incident from my year in London comes suddenly to mind. Somehow, the thing that I remember most from my analysis with Dr. R.——— was when he referred to me, matter of factly, as highly intelligent. Somehow that meant more than all the other erudite insights he offered. I wonder if it shan't be the same with Ginny, in that of all the work I've done with her, most of all she will remember that one day I referred to her as buxom and attractive! She's moved in such an opposite direction from the patient I had screamed at before my last session with Ginny. Ann called to tell me that at least for the time being she would discontinue treatment. I feel that I've really failed with her, but it's with a sense of relief that I view not seeing her again, for awhile. With Ginny, however, I will miss meeting with her next week. I immediately think of my colleague's reaction when I went over some of my reports on Ginny with him a year ago. His first comment was, "You know I think you're a little bit in love with Ginny."

February 1

GINNY

IT'S DIFFICULT to write this report. We talked about my effort to talk to Karl, how it backfired, leaving me feeling anxious. And all the reversals that have happened. My excuses in thinking him strong, unshakable and these being reasons to hide my own weaknesses. Now that we're on the same plane, he as nervous as I, I'm still unable to talk openly and I still feel anxiety and pressure. Perhaps because Karl's anxieties seem like natural reactions to his present situation of having no job, whereas mine seem indigenous. Karl is a healthy person when it comes to the world, to doing things. You chide me saying —are crosswords and racing and gambling healthy? I think they are, making life a game, trying to compete against boredom. Only Karl's lingering physical sicknesses are a sign that he is at war with something. I'm hardly ever physically sick and have had to play the complete nurse to his convalescent self, many times. His sicknesses, whether rooted psychologically or physically, tend to block our lives, and put a shadow over any plans.

The big feeling I got out of yesterday's meeting was that I was unable or unwilling to think about my future. And that I can't answer your questions and don't ask questions of myself.

You told me to work on small things this week. I'll try.

But the haziness of the session has left me maudlin and dopey. (Maybe this has more to do with trying to get unemployment insurance and standing in line day after day.)

It annoyed me that I told you about my friend smoking grass while driving. This preyed on my mind and left me feeling soiled and a traitor. I could tell it was a juicy bit for you and you disapproved. Whenever that happens I always feel a huge generation gap and you become like a parent. Besides it was a throw-away issue. Just trying to make dead-end conversation.

I got this image of someone who is going nowhere and even dawdling at that. That's the way I acted. Fatalistically, I don't like talking about sex either. And since that was a large part of my blabber yesterday, no wonder it bothered me. It seems like using words about it is the wrong medium, and the subject gets squashed and diminished and seems taken care of when it really isn't. It just becomes a black and white porn issue, instead of all the overtones and good things we have in it. Karl and I do some great fluid talking; in fact we engage each other wonderfully and make funny comments and really laugh and are happy. And then the lights go out, and there is no bridge, no dusk between the evening talking and scattering of images and making love, when I somehow feel we are strangers and Karl doesn't want me.

It was comforting when you said I seemed closer than usual to a beginning.

I think I wanted the same responses from you this week that I got last week, you know about being pretty and buxom, and when I didn't get them, I felt I had slid back, that I was flat-chested, figuratively.

February 21

DR. YALOM

A REAL BUMMER. One of the most awkward, strained, unanimated hours I've ever spent with Ginny. It follows my having been out of town for a week and her having cancelled on Friday of last week. She started off saying that it hadn't been a bad two weeks and in fact she had a few days of total well-being. She doesn't know how they started or how they stopped, but she does know that during these times she lost her alienating self-consciousness and was able to write and live with some ease. This morning she woke up hours ahead of time feeling extremely badly. All day she's been anxious, disconcerted, confused and distracted. She said she has a sense of not being able to pull herself together, that people were staring at her on the bus, that she looked like a slob. Somehow I felt that despite the number of things she said, I had little to work with. I naturally chose the subject of her waking early and feeling badly all day, wondering what this had to do with her coming to see me, and got a dearth of information. In fact, there was so little information I was convinced that this was the most important area to investigate.

I put together the picture of Ginny having good times while I was away and then cancelling on Friday when it would have been possible (though a trifle inconvenient) for her to come in. Today she was clearly upset. I asked her whether, in fact, she would prefer not to be here. From this point on things got much worse during the hour. I learned, at the end of the session, that she had mistakenly heard me say that I didn't want her to come anymore. When all else had failed in my attempt to get her working, I tried to make her confront the question of why she continues therapy. What is it she wants to change about herself? No more sure-fire method to evoke anxiety than to pose that question. My analyst in Baltimore, a sweet little old lady, always jolted me with it when I dragged my ass in therapy. Ginny responded that in a few weeks she should be able to come up with a 250-word essay on why she's coming. It was evident that she was angry and things were less warm and more strained between us than before. She remarked that when I took off my glasses and looked at her, my face was just like the face of a lot of other people on the bus. What she meant by this, as I was to find out rather laboriously, was that I wasn't Dr. Yalom so much any more and perhaps less of a friend. Previously she had seen me as a special friend without differentiating me qualitatively from her other friends.

Apparently her change of attitude toward me had been triggered by my suggestion, at our last meeting, that if she really conceived of her major problem as her inability to have an orgasm, she should consider the possibility of specific hypnotic or Masters and Johnson sexual therapy. When I repeated this suggestion today, she was startled to realize that she had virtually dismissed it without considering it at all; so maybe she isn't really interested in therapeutic change.

At one point she said that she doesn't want to have a sexual therapist because it would mean starting with someone else and she doesn't want to do this with me because it would be too embarrassing to deal specifically with that material (although we deal with it all the time). She did point out that, sexually, things are exactly the way they were years ago and that she seems to have made no progress in this area, which makes her feel very bad for not having worked in treatment. I suggested that it must make her feel disappointed with me, since I was supposed to be helping her, but she denied this.

I commented, perhaps a bit snidely, that maybe she was anxious this morning because she must have a symptom when she comes in to see me. She conceded that perhaps she was deliberately trying to make me angry. She knows that anyone would be angry at someone who talked on for an hour the way she was talking. Somehow it was all not very convincing. I was confused about what was happening during the hour and I told her this several times, but we made little headway. It got worse. She replied with several inane statements about her determination to have a good week for me with interesting material for our next session. Things spiraled further downwards and I felt extremely impotent and discouraged.

Well, so much for this dismal session. Ginny's convinced that she brought it with her into the room because she was feeling concentrationless all day long. Perhaps that's so. However, I've been very distracted the whole hour and cannot help recalling that I had another session just like this only a couple of hours ago; so I have to bear at least partial responsibility for this unprofitable hour.

At the end I gave Ginny our reports for the last six months, we will both read them before next week.

February 21

GINNY

OF COURSE with no more discipline than a piece of gum, I read part of your reports before writing my own for the last session.

This will color what could have been the grimness of my report.

When I think back to the session I feel a little angry at both of us. I was angry that you tried to delve into my lifeless anxious mood for so long. I guess quite naturally you tried to find the shoe that fit my aching foot through a multiple choice of reasoning: was I anxious because we had missed two weeks? My sister? Karl? I was your willing associate. As it turned out the mood and feeling were prelude to one of my rare colds, and the Bayer man could have told us and freed us from that topic.

Since I came in already defeated, you talked about therapy not going anywhere. You asked if I thought of it as therapy anymore. I think I said "No" but without thinking. And I suggested that I should write two hundred and fifty words on my goals. Were you more than a friend and if I thought of you as a friend, could we get anywhere?

I read only a few write-ups that night, but it was enough to turn me into lead. I felt so heavy and had to go to bed. It's funny, from your side of the write-ups I get a sense of danger, that all is exposed. From mine, everything is slightly jolly and cryptic and nothing stated simply. Halfway through the week, reading the reports, everything about me seemed so bleak. I felt ashamed. Last week I had accused you mildly of wanting to end therapy. You said I was putting words into your mouth, but when I read the write-ups, it's obvious to me that you are bored and depressed and feel caught up in my own static plunge.

I was not able to concentrate on this too long. Then I remembered a scene with M. J., the encounter group leader. He was speaking to a girl who had had a much more miserable life than I. She had dramatized it beautifully so that we all experienced it almost and were sympathizing. Then M. J. said that she had had twenty miserable years and she was going to have another twenty miserable years, right straight ahead of her. He offered to dance with her and tried to make her laugh, but she held onto that sacred image of miserableness and the old habits. He galavanted around her like a frog, and made her an offer to dance free of pain and her memory. Somehow she saw what she had been doing, an involuntary smile crept on her face, and from then on her life really changed. She made it change. I was still a sponge who seemed never full enough of pity. They told me I was in a hole and would never get out. And I just sat as I do in your office. No jokes were appropriate. And you go with my pace and we lug out together. It would even be fun for me to bring a pack of cards in, and then when we get stuck, we could at least finish gamely.

So this week mechanically I said I would change, force myself. I haven't. Yet somehow I feel more alive.

About sex therapy. In the last two weeks I've thought how nice it would be, but in session I couldn't take the responsibility and come out and ask just what you meant and how to go about it. So I went ring around the rosy. It was like suggesting sex therapy to a three-year-old.

When I want to concentrate the conspiracy inside puts little images that mislead me. Instead of answering your questions I looked at your face and compared it to this guy I hardly know who is attractive with a beard and all. And since you kind of slumped in that chair like a fraternity boy or someone cosy reading a book or drinking beer, I found it easy to digress. If I could have fantasized out loud, something would have happened, but no, I just shop a lot of attitudes and feelings without buying any. And so remain nothing in front of you and me. Like when I saw your sock. I felt like a puppy, like I could get down on all paws and start biting your inside-out sock, and these giddy thoughts cross my adult path every few seconds.

V

A Final Spring

(February 29–May 3)

DR. YALOM

DURING the week Ginny and I read each other's reports. I was feeling somewhat uncomfortable going into the session because although I had set aside a good part of today to read them, some unavoidable circumstances (such as people coming in from out of town) had severely limited my free time and obliged me to skim most of them, especially my own. This was particularly unfortunate, since Ginny had read all the write-ups with extreme care. Unlike the last reading this time she had gone over them several times, and in fact could quote some of the lines.

It was a moving and intense hour for me and I think for Ginny as well. One of the most striking things she did in the session is the very thing she does in her relationship to Karl; she dances away from the stage of real emotions. She avoided both the positive and the negative aspects of her feelings toward me until I pushed her into them. The negative ones came up first; they sprang from my having shown her early write-ups to Madeline Greer, the psychiatric social worker who knows Karl. I of course hastened to explain to Ginny that Madeline hadn't seen any of the reports for over a year; it would have been unthinkable for me to show them to her after I discovered that Madeline knew Karl, nor, for that matter, would Madeline have read them. It was obvious that Ginny was deeply mistrustful and had the right to be profoundly angry at the professional liberty I had taken in sharing her "case material" with another colleague. I think I would have been terribly hurt and angered had this happened to me. Yet she reported to me only a brief flicker of indignation. There was more distrust evident in her statement that she was sorry she had told me about her friend (a sociology graduate student) who smokes a joint every morning because I might use that against him.

She was very much struck by the alternation that occurred in our sessions—after a good one, she would invariably "disappoint" me the next time. She also noted a discrepancy between our respective appraisals of several of the sessions, she feeling good about them while I thought they had gone poorly. She was distressed to discover that

I was much more discouraged and depressed by her than I had led her to believe. I wondered whether or not she wasn't also attuned to some of the positive things I had said, and she acknowledged that by conceding that a few of my comments made her feel very good. It was only bit by bit that we edged into one completely positive section of my notes, and she did this by proffering the idea that I had really revealed more of myself than she had of herself—she was referring to the incident when my colleague had said that maybe I'm a bit in love with Ginny. She slipped gently into the subject by wondering who the analyst was and then by commenting on my courage in being so honest and open. However, she avoided the heart of the matter: the word "love." When I asked her specifically about her reaction to this, she said, with obvious emotion, that she had experienced a feeling of unworthiness and that she genuinely wanted to change for me, now. We discussed her reading the reports at home, where she had to throw them rapidly in a drawer if she heard Karl's footsteps. I observed, as I had months ago, that it sounded like a novel where the heroine frantically thrusts love letters out of sight at the approaching steps of her husband.

Another example of the therapeutic use of the notes hinged on her feelings about publishing them. She talked about this issue, but didn't ask me directly if I intend to publish them. And when I asked her outright why she didn't ask me, she drew herself up with effort in order to frame the question, whereupon I told her that of course I wouldn't without her permission. She then went on to relate some of her fantasies of throwing gasoline on them and burning them in my office, but added that her fears had more to do with the thought of hurting Karl than of revealing herself. She added that she thought my writing had much improved since the last batch. She also asked me if I was seriously considering setting a time limit on therapy, so that she could brace herself for some months of very intensive work. I told her that I wasn't sure but that a logical time would be the end of June, since I am going away for three months in the summer. She skirted the question of termination by asking where I was going, and we never did get very explicit about her feelings of stopping at the end of four more months. Her evasiveness and my own ambivalence have, I suspect, become partners behind our backs.

The last thing she mentioned was a *Sports Illustrated* magazine she had seen in the waiting room with my name on it; she asked whether I read it because Karl did too. I told her that I was interested in sports but that the magazine was more my sons' than my own. Still, I was pleased to have her ask me a question person-to-person. In fact, this was again a session where I felt Ginny to be a grown woman. The grin was gone, she was less embarrassed than I've seen her for awhile, and the vibes were very good between us. She talked about how all the little problems are gone now; she's past the stage of gasoline money, past the poker tantrums, past the incompetent cooking and the cleaning up of tables. Now the bigger issues —her life, her rights, her future with Karl. In fact, for the first time ever, she had the fantasy coming down on the bus today that in the future she and Karl would live in different houses and see each other only for dates. It was also interesting to note that my interpretation about her need to fantasize other people acting unjustly to her so that she might feel righteously angry was very effective in damping those fantasies. She hasn't had them since.

A good, hardworking session, which I end with a feeling of relief because, if truth be told, there was very little I held back in the reports she read. I was being as honest with her as I can think of being with anyone.

February 29

GINNY

NO MATTER WHAT, I did not want a session like last time and prepared myself inwardly to be calm and eager. I started this preparation the night before by reading the reports again, instead of watching T.V. It was a less emotional reading than the first time. I copied down quotes that moved me. I knew that Madeline would be brought up and tried to remember the hot searing feeling I got the first time I read that you were showing them to her. Also I had lost the report I wrote for you. It turns out I had hidden it in my underpants drawer which is so filled with other junk that it got pushed down into the next drawer which is

Karl's underpants drawer. The report of yours had traveled from my underpants to his. I discovered the reports in his drawer today. Thomas Hardy would chuckle at this irony.

Anyway the session started a little late since I waited to be fetched rather than take the initiative at your door. In my own mind I had dressed better than usual. This made me a little self-conscious since I thought you might think I was playing up to you. But it wasn't mentioned and so it passed. I tried to draw first by asking you about the reports. But you won that. We both made the same observations—about the pendulum effect of good and bad sessions. You told me of your disappointment in my holding back both in session and in writing. There is no way for me to answer that. I only have glib muscles; it's all I know how to use. The first layer. It's the contradiction between us since I'm sure I can't get any deeper without tears or emotions. I feel resistant when you expect more than I can give. I feel this whole thing was set up for talking and that the therapy situation with both of us in our leather corners, comfortable, friends, makes it very difficult for me to find my panic. I'm not used to finding my words buried very deep—they are mostly a surface energy and improvisation. I get a hopeless feeling of ever breaking through by just talking and answering questions.

Then we brought up Madeline. You were disappointed again in my distrust of you. That doesn't mean anything to me; I can't take responsibility for initiating a negative feeling and thinking this could really hurt you. So when you tell me I must distrust you, that just glides off my back like water. It doesn't change the way I feel about you. There's no dislike in my distrust. It's something that's over with. I feel discouraged. Because I don't distrust you.

Even though I felt I could look at you in the session, it was to no avail since I didn't have anything new to say.

We brought up limiting the therapy to four months, to come to an end when you go to Europe. This still seems so much in the distance that it doesn't frighten me. I feel so tight and loose at the same time that I can't seem to force myself into making this the most concentrated, important four months and tie all my loose ends together. I see myself going out with a whimper.

When you explained about your colleague and we brought up

the subject of love, I realized how far away I was, cause I felt myself coming back with those words and getting vulnerable again. I titillated myself with a little bit of emotion and sensation, and then stopped.

March 7

DR. YALOM

A CURIOUS HOUR. It began as an arid stroll through the desert—desolate and empty, but in an odd way, pleasantly scented. Eventually the scene of the stroll changed but the fragrance remains and we ended up, I think, feeling very close and deeply engaged. She began with a paradox. First, she had vomited a few minutes ago because she suddenly felt very nauseated on the way up the steps to my office. Second, she'd had a relatively good week. I tracked down the nausea as best as I could, ran into blind alley after blind alley, till finally I was so tired that I was perfectly willing to settle for the lame explanation that it resulted from a free facial which she had had at a cosmetic store in Palo Alto. I made a dutiful attempt to ask why on earth she was having the first facial of her life on the way to see me today (being nobody's fool, I wondered, could it be for me?). No, she daintily demurred in response to my unasked question and proceeded to tell me about the special bargain for facial cosmetics which she had been planning to take advantage of for some time. I tried to find the trail leading into her feelings about stopping therapy in the summer, but we didn't get back to that till later on, at which point it was the key to considerable rich material.

Lots of resistance, but very soft resistance. Ginny told me how good and warm and pleasant she felt, that she wasn't anxious, but that there simply wasn't anything to talk about. Karl's gotten a part-time job. Things are definitely going better for her and him, she tells me almost in passing. She throws out, like a trivial crumb, the fact that sex is now much better between them and that they are having more intimate psychological talks. Sometimes it astounds me the way my patients do this, forgetting all the months and months of work we've done to get to this point, and then as though by the sheerest whim they decide to let me know about the progress they've made.

Then she asks, can she keep coming for four months even if she continues to have nothing to say? I press her for her feelings about ending in June and make it even stronger by saying "only four more months." She denies any strong feelings, imagines how much fun it will be to write me a letter in the future, and indulges in the fantasy of calling on me when she returns to town as a famous woman. There was a lot of emotion tied to this fantasy and her eyes filled with tears; I kept pushing her back into the tears, which seemed to be asking, "Would I take the time to see her?" She said that the fantasy of calling on me filled her with pleasure. Could it really happen? I answered, "What on earth would stop you?" From reading all my notes and knowing me so well, she could have surmised what my response would be. Yes, she realized that.

We spent some time talking once again about her writing. She said that she's really been blocked for about four weeks, has done virtually no writing, and at the same time doesn't miss it too much because her day is pretty full. She misses her writing only when she feels she has nothing important to do and is wasting time, but things have been going well enough with Karl and she finds her life to be pleasantly engrossing. I wondered if I hadn't so aligned myself with the writing that she saw it as mine and not hers. Perhaps she does not write to avoid giving me satisfaction. But I ignored my inner voice and, like the parent of a Hollywood child-star, I suggested we chart out her day and schedule two hours for writing tomorrow morning. Ginny seemed quite receptive. She ended up the hour with a question, which was unusually direct. What would it be like if she were to see me more than once a week? Maybe the week between talks is too long (her previous therapist had said that if she doesn't see her three times a week, it's not worth coming). This makes clear to me how poignant the idea of stopping entirely must be to her. She doesn't let herself really believe that she will stop therapy and always imagines she will see me when I return from my summer vacation. I guess I've handled it the same way because I can't really imagine not seeing her in the future.

March 7

GINNY

IT'S HARD to write anything different about the session from what we comment on while it's still happening.

The important part was when we discussed my feelings instead of random ideas. I felt grounded momentarily. When I think about leaving you I get very sad. And yet I half-played with the idea of stopping session right away and only coming when I have something new to say. I don't know why I said that and then in the same breath I wondered if therapy would change if I could have it twice a week. These were both ways of breaking and tampering with my stronghold against therapy as it has been. It's like you know your husband is going to walk out on you unless you do something.

For once you asked me whether I wanted to continue talking about a certain subject, my nausea. You must have learned from the readings how I sometimes blame you for continuing with hopeless topics.

I got a facial 'cause it was there, as I stumbled through Macy's on the way to your office. And the fragrances and eye liners and lipstick all made me feel slightly sick and in drag.

There's such a difference from when I just tell you things— the boy grabbing me, the cosmetic lady, the haircut, and when I really feel something. It's like I'm there but there's also an interpreter who only translates a third of what is said, ingoing and outgoing. And when he doesn't translate, I can stand at ease (though playing tense). Maybe I feel things will become more acute after therapy is over. And I can be masochistically serene, swooning in my own mischief and fantasy, and head-felt misery. And that now I am too pampered by therapy and comforted by you so even when I feel hopeless about my standing still and driving you to yawn, I end by feeling rejuvenated and happy, being near you, having an audience with you, Papa Yalom. Until the write-up when I force myself into an inward stare and pessimistic forecast. But why do I feel bubbly one moment, and dezone it as something unreal the next moment?

March 15

DR. YALOM

GINNY started off by reassuring me that she has spent time writing yesterday but quickly retracted her "offering" by informing me that it was only a few uninspired scraps. Enough! Enough of this shameless transference, countertransference, minuet. This is the last dance. She cannot be for me the writer I always wanted to be. I must not be for her the mother who lived through her daughter. So I laid it out for us. "Why do you tantalize me with the gifts of your writing? (Why do I allow myself to be tantalized?) Why do you not write during the week instead of regularly waiting till the day before you see me? (Why do I want you to write so much?) Are you writing now only for me? (Why not? I make it clear that this pleases me!)" She did not answer, but no matter, I was speaking as much to myself.

In passing, again, she mentioned a couple of obviously very positive moves. For example, Karl got angry with her and told her that he doesn't want to go out to dinner with her any more, that it's a waste of money and he doesn't see spending money for nothing (this was a day after he had lost $25 gambling). Apparently Ginny held her ground and told him she'd like to go out for dinner. What was the point of her working and making money if she couldn't do the things she wanted to do? And then she left the house and took the dog for a walk. When she came back she had the fantasy that perhaps Karl was going to leave her completely, and much to her surprise (but not to mine) it was quite the opposite, he was solicitous, even apologetic. She seemed puzzled about this and I told her that the more she can oppose him, the more she will be appreciated as a separate person. I said "nobody likes a namby-pamby," my psychiatric adage for the day. We both joked about that. Another incident had to do with their sex life. One evening, sexually stimulated,

Ginny had dressed herself up nicely, but Karl obviously was disinterested in sex that night, which troubled her sufficiently to wake her in the middle of the night. She told Karl what was bothering her and he took it very seriously and discussed it thoroughly with her.

After that she seemed to be really stretching, looking around for things to talk about, and I finally had to say to her that it does actually seem as if she's getting better and for once she had to agree with me. There's no question about the fact that she's feeling more and more comfortable with herself. She said she's disappointed that therapy has to go this way—she had been expecting some miraculous breakthrough full of sound and fury. Her life, even though it is beginning to be more satisfying, has no "mystery." Other people have a secret life, they cheat, have affairs, or adventures; they live dramatically, whereas she has no comparable excitement in her life and furthermore is choiceless, having only one choice in everything she does. I tried to debate that point logically with her. It's quite apparent that she has choices in almost everything she does. She only experiences herself as having no choices. But that didn't take us too far.

Then she talked about her mother's disappointment with her. In her mother's eyes she has no career, no marriage, and no children: so she's a zero across the board. I looked into the subject of marriage and children and nagged her once again to consider whether she wants to get married and wants children and if so, what is she going to do about it? Would she continue with Karl if she were certain he would never provide her with these things? Even though we still had a few minutes to go, she picked up her bag and started to leave. It was clear that I was pushing her too hard, but nonetheless I chided her for not sharing some of her hopes for the future with Karl, since she wants him to share his with her. She has never seriously mentioned to him that she wants children or tried to pin him down about marriage. Perhaps I'm being unwise and unrealistic in expecting her to confront him with marriage and children. Perhaps she is doing it in a much more sensible, well-paced manner. However, she is twenty-seven years old, her childbearing days are almost half over, and I thought I would stir up a bit more anxiety by prodding her on these matters. We'll see next week.

I asked her whether there was anything she wanted to ask me today, just to continue helping her to be assertive. She asked me how I thought the session was going and I told her that I felt things were cozy and comfortable and that she was searching for subjects to talk about. She heard that immediately as a scolding and said that next week she's really going to work hard to find things to work on. She brought up the subject of termination by saying that she was very depressed yesterday (we usually meet on Tuesdays, this week we met on Wednesday because of a committee meeting I had to attend). She wonders if my not seeing her is going to leave a big empty space in her life.

March 15

GINNY

THE MORE tame the session is, the harder it becomes to do the write-ups. For most of the time I was enjoying the things we were saying—what I had said and done to Karl that week. Then at a few minutes to five when I was ready to leave and you gave us some extra minutes, I felt all the good things go down the drain, as you rephrased things that had been happening to me in a different light and I acquiesced. For instance, me having nothing to say about moving, feeling that I had no freedom or secret self, that my writing was boring, etc. I sold myself short. I played the bad things up.

When I got home I realized I had given you ammunition to condemn my mother with (she writes that my letters brighten her somewhat shredded existence). And also by my saying that Karl and I are boring ("an all-time first" you say), I seem to be betraying my relationships. I hate these good guys and bad guys in therapy. That's the way they stack up in my mind. And what's stupid is that I too love letters, that letters brighten up my existence, and that Karl and I are boring, as you and I are boring. Why can't things just be, without seeming bad or wrong?

And then my checklist for my progress:

career
marriage
children

You blame that on my family even though that little test originated in my mind. My mother has never said these things. It's more like an outside appraisal of myself that I give the word "mother" to. But it's unfair. It's me playing the mother. Dampening my day-by-day reality. Of course, the family would like one out of two, or two out of three by the time the bird reaches twenty-seven.

Anyway all of that seemed to happen in the last five minutes when I sunk my anchor again in the muck.

But it felt like a very good day yesterday. Therapy didn't detract. I enjoyed it until I got home.

April 4

DR. YALOM

I HAVEN'T seen Ginny for the past two weeks. One week I was out of town and the second week she cancelled because she was working. She came in a few minutes late, saw me sitting in my chair and meekly asked whether or not she should wait outside. Later she told me how disappointed and limp she felt because she would have liked to have rushed into the room and said with emotion, "Boy, am I glad to see you" or something to that effect. She'd called a couple of times that day without reaching me and my secretary wasn't sure if I were expecting her; so she got on the bus to come in without fully knowing whether I would be here. I gather that on the way she felt a good deal of anger and subsequently guilt about the anger, so that she was almost afraid to see me when she first came in the room.

She immediately, however, launched into her relationship with Karl, which is undergoing a great deal of turmoil. It appears that

Karl has suddenly and drastically changed as a result of an explosive confrontation with Steve, a close friend. Steve sounds like a threatening judgmental person, who came down hard on Karl. They got into a furious argument. Karl was so overcome with anger he ran outside to defuse. He decided to submit, returned to talk in a conciliatory tone to Steve, whereupon Steve fiercely humiliated him all the more. After Steve left, Karl broke down, cried for a while and subsequently became much more willing to examine his feelings. He spent some time talking with a friend, who suggested that Ginny and Karl join an encounter group in Berkeley. Karl, much to Ginny's surprise, was very sympathetic to the idea. As a result of this Karl has been much more open with Ginny; he's been loving, gentle and kind to her and able to say some things that he's never said before. For example, he has let her know now that there were days in the past when he deeply resented her; slowly the whole unspoken substratum of the relationship is becoming available for examination. Ginny is somehow encouraging Karl to do this but, by and large, is not saying a great deal more to him than she has before. At least, so she tells me.

Despite all this rather good news, the session today lacked energy. She seemed tense, a bit withdrawn, somewhat discouraged with herself for not being closer, and I couldn't find any way to stir things up. I had a part in subduing her feelings. There is something about me, I think, which doesn't allow people to express unadulterated joy and enthusiasm.

In the last month she's been working and writing, has had one very good week, two fair ones and one dreadful week in which she went into a tailspin because of a swelling on her cheek which plunged her into cancer fantasies, until a doctor reassured her of its benignancy.

At one point, she asked if I thought she was hopeless. I told her that wasn't my feeling at all, although I wasn't being totally honest, since I was uncomfortable and concerned about the lifelessness between us. She said she felt hopeless because so many good things are happening and yet somehow she's not responding to them emotionally the way she should. Slowly, inexorably, the wheels of change grind on; somehow I play a part in it, at times I'm not sure how, but Ginny bit by bit is slowly changing, slowly evolving and growing. Her relationship with Karl, although I hear it through an unreliable narrator, is obviously deepening and becoming more meaningful.

Then she said she wished she could always be the way she was in M. J.'s encounter group since she was so easily able to play an enthusiastic role there. I agreed that it's easy to play a role on a vacation cruise and she quickly caught my putdown. But she sees as well as I that her role-playing in the encounter group had absolutely no generalizability outside; she remained untouched in her relationship with other people despite a few magic days of real feeling at the beginning.

Some transference material came up to which I didn't know how to respond. When I stood up to get a pipe, she seductively asked, "Would you offer a lady a tiparillo?" Later she mentioned that a friend of hers had written a letter from Germany complaining about the bureaucratic system and life there in general. This seemed relevant to the distance in our relationship and probably to her wish that I wouldn't go to Europe this summer, but she didn't seem eager to pursue my inquiry.

All in all, a kind of disappointing session for me personally, because we remained distant and uninvolved, and yet at the same time I was pleased because she told me good news of changes she's making on the outside.

April 4

GINNY

I HAVE delayed writing this, so see it from an afar of about six days. At the start of the session I thought you looked different, that you were angry or unfriendly. It had been three weeks since our last session but this time you didn't dwell on that.

I was so prepared for you to do me wrong, thinking that you *wouldn't* be there. All afternoon I had interspersed little bits of fantasies with my black and white soda (at the University Creamery). I was conniving in my busy tenth-seeded mind all the possibilities of your not being there, because the therapy day had been postponed. Also on the bus I had just started Sylvia Plath's *The Bell Jar*, which moved me. I was quite willing to suffer vicariously with the heroine of that book. I was more involved with her than with myself.

I don't remember too much of what happened except that at the end, like before, I felt I had betrayed those closest to me.

I filled you in on the previous week and specifically the weekend with the illuminating shocking fight between Karl and Steve and Karl's reactions and how that was changing our life. But there again, I can't believe I do more than get ideas in my head, and never flush them out with emotions or my reactions to things. If ever I had a change to chirp, it was last week when something was finally beginning to happen. But instead of enjoying it fully, I premeditated problems and acted like what had happened was over. You kept insisting that now that the gates of honesty and pain had been opened (by Karl) it would be hard to retreat to our former existence and now was the time to talk to Karl, not just listen, which was good advice—and then you always ask, "Well, what would you like to tell him?" which stumps me. I have a reservoir of faults and weaknesses and I imagine I can't talk without bringing them up, so as usual I couldn't answer you. I feel I have to change a lot for Karl, but right now what I must do for him is be near and listen. I admire the way he lets his emotions run through him. I think he is working on something else, a bigger river than just our relationship. Perhaps his family and other beginnings, which are very twisted and buried in him. It would be moody and selfish of me to ask for some of that action now; besides I think his thoughts will lead to us. The fight has opened up our relationship and made me see new things in Karl that I had only suspected.

I also brought up the bump on my face (bump sounds more tentative than lump). This bump deflates my best times and helps me, depressed, be concave. I guess I did a little hypochondriac thing with you. Always holding myself back. Even if I had gushed out my worst worries, that would have helped. You reassured me a bit by saying there's nothing to worry about in that part of the face.

April 11

DR. YALOM

GINNY started off the session in an unusual way. She read me something she had been writing while she was waiting for me. It was mainly an account of her feelings that day, of what had passed through her mind in a shopping tour, and it was a very touching little vignette which sparkled with bright metaphors. I felt a great deal of pleasure at hearing her read to me and once again I am convinced of her very considerable talent. The other feeling I had, though, was that it was all so frothy, and I wondered if she would ever write about more compelling, larger issues. Here I am, in the vernacular, "laying my trip on Ginny," judging work only by the profundity of the issue which it faces. For the last months I have been deeply engrossed in reading Heidegger just because he deals with the most basic issue of all—the meaning of being—but it's been a terribly self-punitive venture for me since his language and thinking are so agonizingly opaque. Why must I expect others to deal with the same crushing issues?

There were other reasons for her reading this to me aside from simple sharing. In the account, she mentions the fact that she's applying for some jobs, which might make her terminate therapy even more quickly, and she also mentioned that Karl is thinking more seriously of starting therapy. Naturally, irony of ironies, he's thinking of calling Madeline Greer, the one person in the world who has read some of these reports. It would be very awkward, I think, for Madeline to treat Karl, knowing that she has a secret she can't share with him. When I told Ginny these fears, she felt she is getting in the way of Karl's treatment. Obviously, it's all blown out of proportion, because of all the people in the world, why does he have to see Madeline? It's even more absurd in that Madeline is in Palo Alto, whereas there are hundreds of good therapists in the San Francisco area.

Ginny looked very pleasing today, well groomed, with an attractive blouse and long skirt. I also noted that our chairs had been placed rather close together by the cleaning man, and I felt cozy

161

sitting next to her, whereas yesterday with a male patient I felt very uneasy sitting that close to him and moved the chairs away. She talked some more about the bump on her cheek. This time I got up to feel it to see what all the fuss was about, since her doctor now suggested there may be some sort of growth there and I began to get a little alarmed myself that it might be a sinus tumor. It seems like nothing, perhaps an infection of a lacrimal gland. Naturally, however, Ginny has blown it out of all proportion and fantasizes it's a cancer eating away at her face.

She's definitely still very up. Things have gone increasingly well with her and Karl, although they do have their down periods. I tried very hard to make her understand the fact that she's had an up period with him where she's now changed the rules of what can or cannot be talked about and this should give her some strength. And that when things go wrong she really does have the right to say, "Things aren't going as well for us as they were a couple of days ago—let's talk about it." I told her that I wondered what it was that stopped her from saying this to Karl besides "sheer terror." There I am being kind of cute and clever with Ginny and enjoying the pleasure of making her laugh.

We talked about Karl's getting into treatment and how she felt about that, when here she is ready to graduate. She felt a little angry that Karl is just now starting therapy, maybe a bit concerned with all the new demands he'll make on her. She even fantasied that he was standing right outside the door, which is why she was speaking in a whisper. I wondered what it was that he might hear. She said, "Well, if he heard me say that I'm static and won't change as I did a few moments ago, then I think it would be all over." Here again Ginny expressed her sense of the precariousness of the relationship, as if one statement overheard from the person to whom you are obviously deeply committed could cause a total break-up. When I put it in those terms, she could see the absurdity of her statement, but still it isn't very convincing to her.

We did get into one interesting implication of Karl's decision to enter therapy, which is that the therapist will help him see all the negative things about Ginny, just as I in therapy came down heavily on Karl's negative aspects. Thinking about that, I conceded that perhaps Ginny was right. Obviously we did focus on his negative traits because that's what Ginny presented to me as problems, and I never did ask her to talk about the positive things that were going for Karl. When I asked her today, she mentioned some of them. She took it a bit further and pointed out that she's felt all along that I really wanted her to break up with Karl. In a sense, this meant that for quite some time, many, many months in fact, she must have had a sense of somehow defying me by staying with him. This seemed important to me, and I looked into myself and thought about it for a long time. I honestly believe, and told her so, that I never unequivocally wanted her to break up with Karl, but hoped she would be able to make this relationship work to a better extent than it had. (Parenthetically I might add, though I didn't say it to her, if they continue to relate as they are now, then I wouldn't feel too upset if she were to break off with him because she has grown so much that she is capable of other, possibly deeper relationships.) I wanted her to see the distinction between my urging her to leave him and my trying to make her come to terms with the fact that she has the right to leave him. Once she realized that the decision about leaving or staying was hers, as well as Karl's, she would not need to live helplessly under Karl's terrible swift sword which at the moment, at the utterance of one wrong word or the commission of one wrong act, would descend and sever their bond forever.

The last theme was one that has come up over and over again, and I'm not sure how to deal with it. She pointed out how emotionless she is. She would have liked to come in and say in a very animated way that Karl really is going to start therapy and "Can you beat that?" She kept knocking herself for showing so little emotion to me. Now, what am I to do with that? I think, to some extent, her lament has validity in that she still is unusually mild and meek with me. She never loses her temper and often is somewhat childlike. On the other hand, however, I like Ginny quite a bit and if she were doing the other things, it would be playing a role. Much emotion does pass between us and I end up feeling that she is judging herself harshly and unjustly. I keep saying to her, "So what if you had said it in a different way, what would it mean? For me it would only mean that you were playing at something other than what you are." She keeps saying that she's not satisfied with the way she is, that she can't be spontaneous enough. She even brings up failures in spontaneity that she's had in past encounter groups in such a way as to punish herself. I tried to make her realize how terribly insignificant that was, as compared to the real life changes she has been able to make with Karl over these many months, and with me. It all has a circular quality about it, however, because we've been through it so many times. At one point she spoke of a visit with a friend who has a one-and-a-half-year-old child and she is struck by the child's wish that she, Ginny, repeat certain things over and over again. Ginny feels the same way in therapy. There are some things she enjoys saying and some things she enjoys having me do over and over and over again. (Psychotherapy and cyclotherapy.)

Lastly, I tried to bring her to terms with the fact that we really would be stopping in a couple of months. She has never fully accepted this; her fantasy of writing me long letters is just another way of denying the end of therapy and us as "us". I think that in the next sessions I'll have to spend an increasing amount of time on her feelings about terminating, her positive feelings toward me and those that are intertwined with her relationship to Karl, where I am sometimes used to arouse his jealousy. She surprised me by suggesting that I might see the two of them together for a session or two. I think I will do that—it might be a constructive way of aiding termination.

April 11

GINNY

I THOUGHT last week when I told you about Karl wanting help too that you were really taken aback. I might have become a little suspicious about why you should be so adamant against his coming down on a regular basis to see Madeline. "It's so far . . . she's not the only therapist. . . ." It was as if I could be the only prima donna and that was wrong—because right now I'm stable, it's Karl who's hurting, who needs help. I feel guilty too because the only person Karl trusts—Madeline—is ruined for him, in a way. I want Karl to have therapy very much, even though I'm a little scared. I think with both of us in therapy, our life will be less oblivious. I hope Karl will challenge and not just condemn me.

We talked about how I've changed—I keep bringing up this old self and it must be discouraging to you. When you were talking about how I've changed, I thought, why can't I just be happy, why must I "be grabbing at straws" to go back to the past and bring in the encounter groups to show how I've gone down. You like your argument about K and me—that you're not trying to split us up but trying to make me realize that I have the freedom to leave if I wanted, that I could make a choice, and not just be a reflex to something he did. Well, I like my argument too. I feel so confined, I want the freedom not to act the way I do—to be able to have secrets, to be exuberant with no echo chambers, not to always speak to myself and not to always hear myself.

I read the journal to you to impress you, gain your favor, to show what I can do easily, gleefully. It took five minutes away from my shopping.

April 19

DR. YALOM

A WEIRD vaudeville-like hour. Very odd, very puzzling. Ginny comes in and says in a very ebullient way that she'd like to read me a satire she wrote. She then read me a spoof of our last session she had written during the week. It was absolutely hilarious. I burst out laughing as she read it. It was full, however, of references to sexual feelings about me, her need to please me, her need to have me learn from her. I asked her if it would be fair for me to use the content of the satire to help us in the analysis during the rest of the hour. She treated it all in a very giddy, evasive way. We used the word giddy many times and there was indeed a giddy, racy quality. At one point she said she felt like doing back flips for me or a tap dance on my desk. I've never seen her quite this high.

In fact, a lot of good things have happened to her—she's gotten a part-time, well-paying research job for the next four months, where she'll be working with children; she went to the medical clinic, got a complete workup and was given a clean bill of health (the lump on her cheek proved to be of no consequence); she's been writing, with some ease, and things have been going well for her in general.

However, there's a very dark side which is that Karl is obviously becoming more and more distressed. He has been withdrawing from her, having crying spells and moods of despondency during which he's been unwilling to talk to anyone. He has slowly begun to investigate the possibility of getting into treatment. The other thing is that her parents are down, because her sister has had a recurrence of a serious illness.

So in some respects her giddiness and euphoria were impure. My hunch is that though she does admit some superficial feelings of "I should be guilty," she is enjoying the fact that others are suffering while she is on top. At one point she compared herself to a waterbug skimming across the surface of the water quite freely, while others, for example her parents and her sister and Karl, are half submerged, like tin cans floating with their paint peeling off, perhaps even like polluted fish underneath the surface. This was one of the times where I clearly saw what was happening to her and yet opted not to press any interpretation. I felt that I could too easily ignite her guilt and begin a depressive conflagration. It is only too human a thing to feel up when others are down. I think that she and Karl are on a seesaw, where it is not possible for both of them to feel up at the same time. Karl still argues with her and picks at her, but now she needn't take his criticism too seriously; in a sense she's gotten what she wanted for so long—his depression is her guarantee that he will not leave her. Her happiness spills over: she's been turning on the radio when she comes home from work, feels full of life, is seeing her friends, and writing a lot of funny letters. I fear she's probably due for a comedown and will possibly get depressed after this meeting. But in the long run I think she's clearly on an upward trend.

I had a hard time knowing what to do in the hour; to analyze her mirth would have resulted in its dissolution. I tried to explore some of her sexual feelings about me, which were revealed in the satire. No dice. She skittered away, saying that these are just fantasies, that when she starts writing she just lets herself go and they don't necessarily mean much. She wrote the spoof just to demean her feelings and herself. Then she said that she did have some pleasant fantasies about me—if she saw me socially, she would just like to walk with her arm around me and feel close to me.

We talked again about Karl and what she could do to help him. I tried, blandly, to help her realize that maybe this is a time when she could be particularly helpful to him. Perhaps being more open and direct with Karl, even with some of her negative feelings, may be a way of showing real caring. I'm thinking of group meetings for drug addicts, the Synanon Game where gross attack is often called "hard love." She could understand this because one of her friends is doing this very thing to her husband.

Even sexually, things are opening up a bit for her because she was able one morning, recently, to tell Karl that she was almost to the point of orgasm and could reach it, if only he would touch her. He responded to this quite matter of factly by saying, "I can't read your mind, why didn't you tell me?" I tried to underscore the fact that she's taken the difficult first step and should find it easier in the future to tell him what she needs, or better yet, to guide his hand where she wants it to be. She simply wouldn't discuss this with me, under the assumption that talking about it would jinx the whole thing; so I left that too. By the end of the hour I was feeling uncomfortable, not knowing where I could move now that would be helpful to her. I have such mixed feelings. I am very glad to see her looking happier, feeling good, and what's more, I feel that a good deal of it is solidly based, but I have the uneasy feeling that it might all come crashing down very quickly because, for Ginny, good feelings which have their foundations upon others' misfortunes will be evanescent. We shall see.

Ginny's Satire
THE MISFIT

I thought of doing a satire of the session which would be my imagined self that I'm always nagging you with.

Enter bubbling blond, breathless and dying to speak, words spilling all over, like coffee to go. Dr. takes deep breath, waiting for adventure. Devilish look in eye. Girl shows doctor lump on face. Because it's infinitesimal, doctor comes close to touch it—touches girl's face, then neck, then shag. Girl rears up, back arches, with terrific cry explains how she is in her second prime, tells many fantasies of petting with doctor in the happy hour at cocktail bars. Doctor would like to interrupt with questions and interpretations but girl never stops spilling the beans. Through session her face goes from flushed feminine (by Elizabeth Arden) to deathly white, as both love and death rush in her mind. She collapses finally in soft weeping after telling how adoring her boyfriend is becoming, how he wants to open up and buy a massage parlour with her (for a tax loss) and how she doesn't deserve any of it. The doctor tells her she is more buxom even than last week. She hands him her therapy report—five pages, single spaced—every gesture, whimper, thought, dream recorded.

When she leaves, stronger than a thousand facials, she feels relaxed, young. She will be able to leap chores in a single bound. This week she will not be trapped to her kitchen floor, and her table won't be cluttered like a St. Vincent de Paul's. All her silences will be pure. She will advance on the world.

The doctor carries her to the door. He would like to go home to his pot roast, but he daren't. There is so much to write. His memory is ignited. He has learned so much, too much from the girl.

She walks past Stanford's grave and the spring sun squints at her from every tree. She feels at one with the cacti, and the palm.

Once on the Greyhound bus her strong face keeps away all of the Third World who are traveling the bus. Go Greyhound and leave the minorities to us. She takes a whole seat and falls asleep. Her dreams, like dictaphone machines, play back her doctor's voice and touch. As the bus speeds away, she vows in her mind to dedicate all her books "to her doctor." And then so people will not think it is to her chiropodist or her gynecologist, she sings, "to Dr. Y. who gave me the freedom to cry, the oomph to fly, and ten reasons not to die."

Written by Ms. Fits

April 19

GINNY

I THOUGHT yesterday we were just like two friends getting together. Except that only I talked about my problems. I really was happy and would have been more at ease if it weren't supposed to be therapy. I loved the way you laughed at the piece I wrote. Then of course you wanted to know if it were fair to use it as evidence, as incentive for the session. And I cut you off from doing what you wanted to. What I had written was a larger than life caricature and by it I both exposed and protected myself. I was also horribly sarcastic, which is the easiest way for me to be. Only later riding the bus home I thought I might have disappointed you, by tantalizing you with it, then stopping discussion.

I tried to draw off some of my energy in the session, thinking of Karl and feeling guilty. None of this was emotional though. Maybe because I don't really feel guilty; I even welcome what is happening in order to help us.

Part of me judges the whole session as superficial. But the part that laughs and relaxes enjoys it immensely.

I never thought of myself as ebullient yesterday until you brought it up. By the end of the session, though, I was going stale. I'm too lazy to struggle after something, to find a straight path and keep after it. Instead I succumb to the old wraps to cover myself up in.

April 23

DR. YALOM

ONE OF the dullest hours I've ever spent. The minutes stretched out interminably. Suddenly it was as though there was absolutely nothing for us to talk about. It was as if Ginny had rummaged

169

through all of our interviews of the past year, picked out the most tedious parts of each, rolled them into a big ball and bounced it for an hour in my office today. I wasn't feeling too well, having had a bad night's sleep, and I kept wondering if it was me. But I don't think so. I had a great deal going on today and was pretty much up to everything else. She simply didn't bring up any issue we could work on, nor could I find any way to help her discuss anything. In fact, she came in and said straight off that she didn't know what she was going to talk about, she had thought about it but gave up and finally decided not to plan anything. I suggested we take a look at the calendar and make up our schedule; it turned out that we have about eight more sessions left. She wanted some assurance that she could see me in the fall just to review the summer, and also that she could write me in Europe, and then also asked jokingly whether she could trade some of the interviews in June for some in September. I told her that I'd like to see her in September, but only to review the summer. I tried to make it clear that June is "termination."

Then she said that Karl had started therapy and it looks as if it is going to be helpful. She wonders if she shan't be jealous of all the attention Karl will get; perhaps she will have to manufacture some convincing complaints. After that, a large frothy nothing. Every time she mentioned something and I tried to get hold of it, there was just nothing there. The happiness she felt at the last session lasted for several days. She knows she should use our remaining time for something useful. Her friends tell her that she should come to terms with her mother and father. O.K., so I try to go into what "coming to terms" means. She doesn't have any idea. The more I press, the more I realize that there is nothing to be gained. She has a friend who is going to several encounter groups and is really "learning who he is." I tried to explore that with her, but she recognizes the encounter group "highs" as something no longer useful for her. She talked about not responding to some insults Karl had thrown her way—stale and non-nutritious material. She talked about her feeling that she should be doing more in life, taking advantage of her opportunities, sitting straighter. . . . I no longer know what the hell she is talking about and I try to confront all the "shoulds" that she carries around with her, wondering if those aren't in fact her mother's voice.

I guess I'd like to hear her say that everything is really going well, for my own reassurance. To the best of my judgment, though, things do go well, so well that she has to struggle hard to keep on being able to present herself as a patient. There are only a few minor discontented areas, such as her inability to oppose Karl on some occasions and also a few disturbing dreams, one of them having a lesbian theme. But I've never worked much on dreams with Ginny because she hides behind them and I'm trying to find Ginny, not understand her. At this stage of therapy I could see the dream she presented for what it was: a Lorelei beckoning me into therapy without end. I simply closed my ears and told her she's always going to have dreams like this—it's a part of being human. I'm not quite sure what I wanted her to talk about. Maybe, we really are finished and I'm dragging it out too long. At any rate, I'm sure she'll have a real downer from this interview. I'm left already with a rather bad taste in my mouth. I feel that I did nothing to help her; everything I tried was halfhearted because I seemed to know in advance that it wasn't going to be much help.

April 23

GINNY

I'VE GOTTEN the session mixed up by the night that followed. Rather the night drained any of the fun out of the session. I woke the next morning hating you. The way I've been in the session—flippant, gay, mushy, not at all sure inside how anything was going, asking you to find out; not bringing up new things, acquiescing, saying yes I was happy, yes I was sad, being anecdotal rather than emotional, a puppet state.

Anyway that night all my worst fears poured out. K asked why I was so timid with him, afraid to talk to him, and if I were so afraid, how had I stayed with him so long? These are obvious things I always thought inside myself but you told me I was chiding myself for nothing. The same horribly stagnant quality in me these last months in session had not gone unnoticed. As in session, I can't say anything to him without playing it first inside my mind, with a whole background of canned voices and derision. In session when I droop and you say, "What are you thinking?" then my head bobs up, I grin and say something. And this is progress? You should have kicked me in the head or thrown me out. I would rather have suffered from you, tested out my pain with you, whom I'm not sharing all my feelings, furniture and food with. I would rather have stood up to that, as a test case, then have to drown now, at night. The first hint of silence, of criticism, of need on K's part, and the most overwhelming fear explodes and it feels like an anchor that sinks, holding me dead for eight hours. I'm not able to sleep, I imagine the worst corners of my fate, I lavishly fantasize even while the thing is happening and something is being asked of me. I hate every redeeming feature that makes me survive in the day. I join hands with the worst Ginny of college board nights, of any test that demanded something from me.

Anyway I held off writing this cause it had nothing to do with you or the session and is or should be directed against me. You are only an accessory, having shared our little bubbling hour.

I forgot what we talked about in session. I asked you how you would change me, this was filler material. You said I could be more assertive. Oh yes, you said it was so hard for me to think of anything wrong. What a joke.

May 3

DR. YALOM

ONE UP one down. Ginny really is right, the sessions do alternate strikingly in their meaningfulness. This was an odd session in which I felt both busy (by which I mean that I was doing whatever it is I am supposed to be doing with people: I was working because I had something into which I could sink my teeth) and, on the other hand, genuinely despairing for Ginny. I couldn't avoid the feeling that perhaps nothing has really changed after all, that perhaps she's just as fucked up as she always was, that perhaps the behaviorists are right and I should just try to deal with her behavior, giving her instructions on how to change and how to behave. A feeling that it's all too overwhelming persisted for the first 15 to 20 minutes, but then gradually things began to make more sense.

The crucial event for today's session occurred last week right after our last meeting. That night when Ginny was in bed with Karl, he asked, "Ginny, why are you afraid of me?" Apparently she handled that situation very badly. She couldn't answer him, he kept pressing her, she ended up feeling like a terrible failure, and things grew worse and worse. Well, I had many thoughts about this, almost all of which I shared with her. First I said that here was the long-awaited invitation. She's always lamented how impossible it was for her and Karl to really talk, that she's always had to sit on her fear and her feelings because Karl wanted it that way, and here he had finally offered an unequivocal invitation to open verbal discourse. I tried to role play it with her, giving her suggestions as to what she might have answered; I tried to help her formulate what it was she really feared. What was this terror that paralyzed and muted her? She answered that she was afraid he would leave her; but because he's so critical of every little thing that she does, she is also frightened of his presence. In the role playing I reinforced almost every statement she made. Almost any utterance is better than mutism, better than being the blob or shadow which I imagine she must be so often to him. Perhaps I was too hard on her but I kept trying to make her see that she's got so much to say which Karl wants to hear, but I don't think I came across in the most supportive way. I asked her whether she wanted to continue role playing or to talk about why she is afraid of me, the latter being closer to a real life situation. She said she'd rather do that, so I asked her why she was afraid of me; was it because I must get sick of her at times for not changing, or for being the way she was last week? Did she feel after last week that something bad was going to happen, that I'd punish her for not taking anything seriously? I admitted that at times I am disgusted, like last week, but that is not my overall feeling.

I then made an interpretation to her, which I think is probably true; by continuing to fail with Karl she's attempting magically to keep me at her side. She refuses to grow, refuses to change, and it's a reaction to our impending termination. She smiled and said, "I knew you'd say that." But we couldn't take it very far. We also considered whether she wants to drive Karl away. I gave her some specific instructions as to how she could respond to him when he criticizes her. Why does he have to be so critical of her, in general? Why is it that she can never be critical of him? I asked her what she'd like to say when he complains about her incorrect way of washing the dishes. She said, well, sometimes she'd like to say "fuck off." I told her that if I were he, I'd much rather hear that than nothing at all. So once more, in the endless revolving sequence of cyclotherapy, I gave Ginny a pep talk and sent her back into the ring with huge pillows of boxing gloves on. She does make me feel that she is so helpless.

I suggested to her that she should think seriously of bringing Karl into the office next week. She's indicated that she may very well do it, if he's willing. That would be a fascinating hour!

May 3

GINNY

THE SESSION was helpful to me. You took a more active part. After I told you about the fiasco of Karl asking me why I was afraid, we role played. When Karl asked me, I froze, and whatever I thought of, didn't say. I was on remote control, too busy eating away at myself to do anything to help.

But this time magically when you asked why I was afraid, the sentence was allowed to touch me. The way I know is I stop gabbing inside and have a blank moment in my head, and something better takes hold of me. You gave me confidence that anything I said to Karl's question could be an answer, as long as I spoke and didn't bury it.

I didn't know that you would think I rigged up the fiasco to show I did need therapy and you. But when I thought about it, it seems just like what you would think of. I think for once you're wrong. I have a bad habit of not speaking clearly. Of getting lost. This whole time in therapy has been like a giddy detour, with me the one not wanting to find the right road. I couldn't answer Karl; I usually don't answer you. I feel better. I don't want to be pounced on. If I had succeeded more with you, I would have with Karl and vice versa. It's not because I want to keep the stalemate we've had that I so often fail.

When you told me how you felt about the session before—that it was "disgusting"—it made a big impact. Not at the moment (then I thought it was cute). But since, I've been thinking of it ("disgusting" it makes me feel bad). I only think of myself. What myself thinks someone else is thinking, if I could know your reactions instead of imagining them. And I know what you'll say: "ask."

To take away part of the guilt for subjecting you to my bouts, of course, I fantasized writing a journal for you this summer. It would be better than the write-ups. And in giving it to you in the fall, I would have to see you at least once. The fantasy deteriorates. I think how I would have to roast other people in talking about them. And I'm glad I don't have to write it.

I can't remember whose suggestion it was to bring Karl. A good guess would be yours. A very generous offer. I thought at the time it would be wonderful. When you think how scared I used to be of that, you see how far you had inspired me yesterday. Then you made a joke of my worst fears—a shotgun session with you asking Karl when he intends to marry me. It's funny when V. (previous therapist) had a session with my parents and me, I didn't say a word. I was like a little deity with her picture on the wall. One was conscious I was there, glowing, rooting for both sides against me in the middle.

When I got home I thought I have only about four sessions left. I couldn't bear to waste one, to share one, to play the spotless ingenue again when I've gone a few slippers beyond that. If Karl comes, I want it to be really good.

I'll feel like a martyr who sacrifices a session because it is the right thing to do. But I really dream about a good session with the three of us.

VI

---

*Every Day Gets
a Little Closer*

(May 10–June 21)

DR. YALOM

ENTER THE WORLD. Something very different happened today. Ginny brought Karl with her. I had been very tired all day, having slept little the night before, and therefore ambled somewhat drowsily into the waiting room to collect Ginny and bring her into my office. Suddenly I see this man sitting next to her, and it dawns on me that this must be Karl. At the end of last session I had seriously suggested that she bring him, but as she had never taken up similar offers in the past, it never really occurred to me that she might have the courage to issue the invitation and that Karl might accept. Whenever we had previously considered such a move, Ginny had not thought Karl would be willing to entertain the idea. At any rate, there he was. My fatigue and drowsiness rapidly vanished and I rode a keen wave of interest the whole hour. In fact, it was one of the most interesting hours I've spent for a long, long time.

Karl was so different from what I had anticipated. With considerable certainty I had envisioned him as a dark-haired, gruff, heavily bearded individual, who would be closed or challenging or hostile to me. Instead, he was quite the opposite, delightfully open, free, courteous—an extremely handsome blond man with long straight hair. Ginny was well dressed and well groomed, and I experienced a great deal of pleasure at being together with these two terribly attractive people who, despite everything else they had to say, obviously have warm, tender feelings for each other. At times during the interview I felt little pangs of jealousy, for I had always considered Ginny mine, and suddenly I see what a really distorted illusion that has been. She's been so much more Karl's than mine. He lives with her all day long, he sleeps with her at night, and I have her for a single hour a week. But these are only passing thoughts. I was very interested in Karl and he did most of the talking. With a marked self-assurance at the beginning of the session, as I was sipping a cup of coffee, he asked whether he could have one too. I realized that I had been remiss in not offering him one and ushered him into the coffee room, where he, with considerable aplomb, helped himself.

I started off by suggesting that we consider the problems that exist between the two of them, and fairly soon we got into a very constructive use of time. With refreshing openness Karl discussed his annoyance at Ginny's failings—the badly washed dishes, the badly cooked dinners, etc. He wishes she were more competent and more effective. Ginny countered with the assertion that the kitchen was spotless today, and then Karl passed on to a somewhat higher level of demand—that she be able to tackle problems in the outside world. I gradually heard very clearly something Ginny has been saying that I haven't been fully appreciating, which is that Karl is really telling her: "Be something other than what you are. Be different. In fact, be just like me." I bided my time and finally implied as much to Karl. I wanted to say it gently so that he wouldn't feel attacked, for I imagine he must feel like an uncomfortable outsider here with me and Ginny who have spent so much time together. However, he accepted my interpretation very, very easily. Later on, we were able to conclude that not only did he have clear ideals for Ginny, which he elaborated explicitly, but that he had some very strong ideals for himself, and he responded most vigorously when he spotted certain traits in her which he disliked in himself. He dislikes her docility and her passivity and certainly he abhors any traces of these traits in himself.

I was proud of Ginny today. She kept speaking up, talking back to Karl, she even brought up the issue of his leaving her, but she said it so quickly that it was almost passed over. I was reluctant to pick it up since we were too near the end of the hour for something as loaded as that. She revealed how frightened she was of him and he confessed that he makes her frightened, perhaps even intentionally. He was quick; he easily understood that there is a price to be paid for having his own standards for Ginny—she will squelch parts of herself which he would like to see. I think this was a very important insight for Karl—he heard it and, I believe, allowed it to register.

Karl is not a closed, defensive person, and I should imagine he could work well in therapy. Apparently he has some severe identity problems and a relentless drive to be the person he thinks his parents expect him to be. He has much therapeutic work ahead but considerable ego strength.

I am curious to see Ginny's next write-up, for I wonder what this meeting meant to her in terms of transference toward me and in terms of her feelings about me vis-à-vis Karl. Somehow I've always underestimated Karl, never appreciated him and never understood what a potentially good thing Ginny has going for her, and conversely, I can see how attractive Ginny is in so many ways to Karl.

At the end of the hour, I tried to confirm my feeling that the session had been a constructive one by asking if they were able to talk as freely as this at other times. (Will I never stop needing applause?) Of course, they said no, they are talking much more freely now. I tried to extend this into the future to keep the new options open by asking Ginny whether she may henceforth be able to tell Karl when she feels somewhat squelched by him. She said she thought she could.

May 10

GINNY

IT WAS so funny to see you round the corner ready to welcome me, and then get surprised by seeing Karl.

Naturally I had not thought about what was going to happen, ignoring the inevitable. I was proud of both of you. And my silences sometimes seemed like indictments against me, so I jabbered.

I learned a great deal. There was a moment when I seemed to understand my behavior toward Karl. I never imagined Karl was so dissatisfied as he said. And later I mulled over this to distraction and anger. I saw how I had webbed myself in groceries, cooking and cleaning or recriminations about not cleaning, and that this full-time pastime wasn't appreciated at all. Of course I know that in therapy I always exaggerated and tended to overstate the case and maybe Karl, in the luxury of an audience, exaggerated too.

You kept emphasizing how one-sided things were with Karl wielding all the criticism toward me. All my feelings were responses toward something he had once thought about me. All his goals were him and all mine were us.

I never thought that Karl might inhibit me, but maybe that's true. I think you were wrong suggesting I deliberately leave a glass dirty so as to hit him where it hurts. Of course, I've always irked people by doing things only half-way, not following through. I fade, though unintentionally. I take half breaths, never fully exhaling.

After the session we were alive with all that had been brought up. And as we elaborated on what had been said some of my buoyance was caught up in an awful undertow. Karl felt that my being so afraid of his leaving was what hemmed him in; that I would fall apart. He wanted me to have my own life. He thought this weakness was the most despicable part of me. He wants me to get my own life and I almost finished the sentence —so he will not be afraid to leave me.

The tables were turned. I had always thought I was protecting you from Karl's abuse. But he thought you were wonderful, intelligent. I almost plotzed when he expressed a wish that he should come back. He thought it was weak of me to have considered not taking him.

I really enjoyed it and was grateful to you. You seemed to be my true friend.

May 10

KARL

I HAD no real idea what to expect, although, having just started therapy in a group, some of the nervousness that I might have felt was allayed. Still, I felt like I was entering some new territory which I couldn't quite see, and had never quite seen, and maybe now I was going to find out if it was really there. Just after we went into your office I saw your coffee and asked for some; I think I wanted time to get my bearings more than the coffee.

We ended up sitting in that triangle arrangement, with you at the apex since you were against the shorter wall. I wondered if I shouldn't be sitting next to Ginny or she next to me, but soon became glad that we were across the room from each other. It made me able to talk more freely and I felt very comfortable exactly that far away from both of you. I had room to move and whatever I said, even something that had not been said before, didn't seem to be aimed at you or Ginny but more like pushed in a big ball of words across the space which gave her time to prepare to receive it.

My fear was that we would get sidetracked, trying to shove our larger emotions into the boxes of our smaller points of annoyance, which had been happening in the therapy group and had been leaving me feeling unconnected with them, brittle, a little hysterical over not much. But when I began to talk, I felt like it was coming from the core and that what I was saying was exactly what I felt. At times I wondered why I hadn't been able to say it before. Your few comments always helped to nudge us into the unexplored corners. I think some of my ease came from my discovering that it wasn't going to be Ginny and you, who knew more about me from Ginny than I knew about me from Ginny, against me. I had decided that I would not fight if that came about since I had had many of my self-confidences shattered recently with the results being good; but the thought of our hour of shock and bewilderment and of the next few days or however long it would take to work through it again wasn't appealing. When I saw that wasn't going to happen, I felt like giving.

I worried from time to time that I was talking too much but I was also worried that I might not be able to say those important things in just that way again. I am still worried that I am not the listener I once was. I had always assumed that if I withdrew and shut people off, they would hammer to get in; instead, I think they often just shut *you* out. But during the session I was sure I was being heard and it almost made me drunk.

On the other hand, I find that in writing this I am more fascinated with my own responses and motivations than I am with considerations of how Ginny feels or felt about it all and I suppose somehow and someday I am going to have to face the questions of whether that is how I treat people or whether that is how I would treat any lover or whether that is how I treat Ginny alone.

If it should turn out to be the latter and if that meant that I should leave her, it would be very difficult for two paradoxical reasons. On the one hand, I would have a kind of horror at having to face life alone again, but on the other hand, I feel trapped because I think my leaving Ginny would crush her, that after this time together and letting her build her days around me it would be abominably cruel for me to leave her alone. I would be afraid for her sake to leave for my sake and so I pull back and forth in a room where I am growing restless; at the same time I am afraid of what I would find on the other side of the door—at least the room is familiar and often reassuring—and afraid of what would happen in the room when I had left. Some of this Ginny and I talked about after we left your office, but I'm not sure what to do. Often when she annoys me I think, right at the time too, that I am judging her on superficial values that I should have outgrown by now. I tell myself that I feel what I feel because she does not fit a high school pattern of coolness that I haven't shaken off, though it seems unworthy of her and me; and I don't know enough about myself or about life to tell whether what I am seeing in all that rough is a diamond or a few glints of sunshine off a piece of glass.

May 24

DR. YALOM

AFTER the last session I wasn't quite sure whether to expect Ginny alone or Ginny and Karl today, but they both appeared again and, surprisingly enough, Karl handed me a long write-up, which I hadn't asked for. Ginny rather apologetically pointed out that hers was all soggy and messy and has yet to be typed. She seemed to be unusually ill at ease and unable to decide whether she should give it to me or not. This opening gambit turned out to be an accurate predictor of her behavior the rest of the meeting.

We started off by Ginny saying that the last interview had been very good and enjoyable during the session and that they had done a tremendous amount of talking afterward. She's not sure what other repercussions resulted from our meeting, but she knows they have been talking more and fighting more. In response to my question about the content of these discussions, we moved fairly quickly into some important material. Most of the discussion was between Karl and me, with Ginny remaining largely on the sidelines. She explained some time later that she was feeling tired and somewhat out of things, because she'd had her eyes dilated that day and also because she's gotten a new job. That wasn't the whole story.

Karl immediately tackled the issue of his being afraid to leave Ginny because she might fall apart. If ever there was a core subject for a couple, this was it—Ginny and I have on so many different occasions debated why she could not talk with Karl about the future of their relationship. It was a compelling experience to sit there and hear them discuss something so matter of factly that Ginny had been dreading to bring up for month after month after month. Karl feared Ginny would be depressed and go to pieces if he were to leave her, and that he would subsequently be overwhelmed with guilt when he realized what he had done to her. I asked about the effects on him and he admitted fearing the same thing for himself; he's never enjoyed living alone and he's not sure whether he wants to. He is, however, tempted by the challenge, feeling that it's somehow a failing for him never to have been able to succeed in being entirely self-sufficient. To my way of thinking, living together because they are afraid to live apart is a meager basis for a relationship and I said so. It's hard to imagine anything enduring which is built on so insubstantial a foundation.

Throughout the session I kept trying to encourage Ginny to speak up, so that Karl would know what she was thinking and be less obliged to read her mind. A good example of this occurred in a long argument they had recently, too detailed to go into here, but which consisted of Ginny's wanting to go out with friends, Karl's refusing and then consenting to go out anyway when he noticed by Ginny's long face that she was terribly upset. They both ended up having a bad time. Was it not possible for them to learn explicitly from each other how important the occasion was for each of them and then make a joint decision which would somehow make room for their respective needs? (Easier said than done, said I to myself, as I reflected upon comparable debacles with my wife.)

I suggested that Ginny may have some investment in appearing fragile since it is one way of keeping Karl bound to her. Obviously she didn't enjoy my saying that. In fact, it's similar to the interpretation I've often made to her about her relationship with me, i.e., that she has to remain sick in order to keep me. At one point in the session she showed a not-so-fragile, almost hearty Ginny by vehemently refuting one of Karl's statements. When he said that she had no understanding of how important a certain article he was writing was to him, she flashed back almost fiercely, "how do you know?" and went on to demonstrate that she was fully aware of his feeling and had tried, though ineffectively, to convey to him her own concern about the article. Having so often prompted Ginny from behind the scene, I found it thoroughly satisfying to watch her defend herself.

Karl then returned to the theme of Ginny's incompetence. He cited an example of a recent party where Ginny had appeared very foolish because she didn't understand a joke that everyone else obviously understood. In my office Ginny was painfully embarrassed—she didn't quite know why she had misinterpreted the joke. Furthermore, Karl felt very embarrassed. In fact, all three of us were caught together in a tangle of embarrassment. I didn't know how to turn this awkward scene into something constructive, except by pointing out that all the demands for change were very unidirectional; Karl makes many demands for Ginny to change but she never makes comparable demands of him. She said that what she'd really like to change in Karl is his constant criticism of her, which makes for a mind-boggling Gordian knot. Karl looked embarrassed and he was; I tried to find out why. I think he is just beginning to sense that his demands on Ginny were unrealistic and unfair. But we didn't really get too far into that.

I wondered about Ginny's inability to criticize Karl, whereupon they both agreed that, until two or three months ago, Karl was virtually unassailable. In fact, had she criticized him, he would have become irrationally angry. Therefore, only an obsequious, self-effacing Ginny could have stayed with him. I wondered also whether her so-called incompetence wasn't somehow a function of her inability to criticize him openly and whether the only form of retaliation available to her wasn't a passive aggressive one—continuing to do the little things that pissed him off. Karl really dug that interpretation because it supported what he had always believed—that

Ginny could, if she wanted to, do the household chores. Ginny received the interpretation with a wan, sickly smile. All in all, I think she was unnerved by the session. I tried to check it out at the end of the hour by asking if she felt picked on by the two men who seemed to be hitting it off so well. Did she feel a bit left out of the triangle? She evaded me and my question, and at the end of the meeting seemed to slink out of the office. Karl, on the other hand, thanked me heartily and shook my hand.

Although I didn't leave the session with a very good feeling (I let it run over ten minutes in a vain attempt to recoup some of last week's vigor), it is clear that these meetings have changed something for the better between the two of them: they will no longer be so distant and closed and obliged to resort to mind reading and guesswork. Some rules of the relationship are now permanently altered. We agreed to meet as a couple for the next two sessions and then Ginny would have the last two sessions to herself. I wish that I had started seeing the two of them together quite some time ago. Everything is moving quicker now.

May 24

GINNY

I GUESS I let Karl do most of the talking. I was feeling very tired, pre-migraine, and became full-fledged migraine by the evening. Some of what I said seemed to come out of nowhere (like telling you I had started work) but I was confused and didn't know how to share the session.

You seem so much more directive in these sessions, initiating questions, summing up. Of course Karl supplies you with a lot more information than I ever did.

I thought it was funny that one of my prime fantasies (being alone, living alone) should be Karl's too. It's a kind of unrealistic stake to compare our so much shared existence to. And to berate our respective weaknesses in needing someone. Listening

187

to Karl tell it, I could identify and see how it is an easy pasture to let your imagination go wild in.

Karl didn't think that I would be the one to leave, which coincided with my own appraisal. I used to talk to you and you'd say, "Well, why couldn't you be the one to leave?"

It seems like the major time I was in therapy with you, my home life was stuck and static, Karl and I both tacitly in limbo, a little wounded and trying to heal.

Karl also seemed to go through the same thing I did in therapy, being full of doubt as to the value of our relationship, to the point where the overwhelming verdict seemed to be to get out, and yet we both try to avoid that direction, because basically we like each other. I was touched by his diamond/milk bottle dilemma. Which one am I? With all these cartons I guess a real glass milk bottle has some value.

The session seemed to touch mildly on important, crucial issues but it was as if we were predisposed to be kind to each other and just look at old on-going wounds without trying to open them to infection.

I wanted ten minutes alone with you. For Karl and I had talked about sex during the past two weeks with a little breakthrough. But I felt I couldn't bring this up at the session. I was like a creaky hinge on the door of conspiracy. You were most constructive when you asked us to explore how we let each other know how we feel. I think we all maintained a sense of humor. I was surprised to learn that Karl thought I wasn't interested in his writing. I thought I had shown great, constructive interest. It's true at a certain point he changed his writing style, abandoning a personal, evocative one for a more professional abstract one (writing more for a commercial market—*Playboy*, no less), and I favored the first, because I am really starving for glimpses into Karl's family and memory and I think the more personal writing about his childhood and adolescence helped him to feel his imagination and its neglected content. That night some of my friends called, interrupting Karl's writing silence; I was unaware my popularity with Karl had plummeted, that he was furious, taking it as a sign I did not care about his writing because I didn't tell my friends not to call me. I would fight back if only I knew I was being silently attacked.

Since the last two sessions I'm more able to stand up for myself because I see that Karl does take things seriously and is constantly making judgments about me; that my evasions and silences are not just blank spots but big black marks against me. Just the fact of going here together makes us feel much closer. And we're more caring in everything—fights, talks, etc.

I only wish this had started earlier so that I could have had my cake and eat it too. And be close with each of you.

May 24

KARL

THE SECOND time I think I felt over confident and wanted a rerun of the week before, which had accomplished so much. I was less aware of you as a presence and felt myself to be on the center of the stage, which is where I usually try to move when I start feeling sure of myself in a situation. However, I found that I couldn't speak so closely to my feelings and that the discussion kept getting sidetracked and issues manufactured since we were with a therapist; that is the tone of discussions with some of our friends whom Ginny likes and I don't. On the other hand, the best things that came out of the session seemed to go very deep—I am thinking particularly of your suggestion that Ginny continues a kind of sloppiness about the kitchen, etc., as a protest against values I judge her by, but which she doesn't hold herself; while, at the same time, she is afraid to confront me directly. Although that sentence is confused, I did get the point.

I don't think I have learned what to expect from other people. Last night I came home about eleven after playing cards. I was disgusted with myself for going to the game since I had work to do and it was a night I could have had with Ginny. I was afraid of backsliding. We talked for several hours and I began to feel more comfortable and at ease and had renewed confidence that I could do what I want to do. Without Ginny, I would have spent the night brooding and growing more convinced of my purposelessness and ultimate failure. I told her all this, too, which was really like icing on a cake. Where had I been all these years, I asked myself? Why had I never seen that comfort and sharing was something to value and something that would not exist without her? Since I am just starting to realize what Ginny can do for me, I have only just started to realize what I can do for her.

I think that's really all I have to say because what I have talked about so far has been of great moment. I don't quite know what to add. You will see me only one time and Ginny only twice more and I suppose you might be interested in the relation between our meetings and what is happening between Ginny and me. I can't be really sure since I am still so close to all of it and want to stay that way for a while. I think I was lucky to get to see you when I did since it was at a crucial time for us, but it was also at a time when I was ready to hear what I might have been afraid to listen to before. I also think that what happened in the first visit enabled me to see that problems could be solved and the second session helped isolate some of the problems. One other thing: in the second session I became worried about boring you when the discussion would drift to what I myself found boring. I was amazed when you would choose exactly those things—say the dirty dishes—to press. Later I decided that I might be consistently using boredom as a defense. There are things that *do* bore me; but it can also be a convenient mechanism for keeping myself blind to what I should or could see.

Would the progress that has been made have happened anyway without our meeting? I don't know. I don't think it would have happened so quickly since you acted as a catalyst that got me to relax enough to confide in Ginny.

I think that's all I can say right now.

May 31

DR. YALOM

I'VE BEEN in this business for a long time, but the interview today represented one of my peak experiences as a therapist. I felt so happy that I was near tears on a couple of occasions. It was so good, for once, to see the fruits of long and very hard labor. Maybe I'm exaggerating in a spirit of self-aggrandizement, but I don't think so. I kept remembering all the time and effort I've spent seeing Ginny and also all the hard work that she's done over all these months. Everything seems to have been pointing toward today, and everything fell into place—all the issues that Ginny had talked about with me, all the fears that were so irrational, all the things that she was afraid to say, afraid to bring up, afraid to face, she faced today in the session and has faced on her own with Karl during the past seven days. When I think of all we've gone through and now how quickly we are moving, I begin to believe once again in my work, in the slow, sometimes intolerably slow, business of building firmly and well.

They both came in feeling very, very good about one another, saying they had spent much time over the weekend talking together in a way they never had before. They aired their respective feelings about Karl's leaving, about Ginny's fear of Karl, and so many other unspoken, crucial matters, which brought them very close to one another. Karl said that suddenly the house felt different to him, that it was one of the first times in his life that he really wanted to be with and close to someone. And so the first part of the session was a kind of testimonial banquet. I basked. And then I wondered aloud whether we should rest on our laurels or move into new areas. Neither of them could think of anything else they wanted to discuss. Secretly I wanted Ginny to bring up something she has never dared to mention to Karl—her night panics when she is full of terror and afraid to give expression to her sexual needs. Delicately I hinted to her to venture into this sensitive area, pointing out that it was hard for me to bring up certain issues because I feared I might be breaking confidentiality. She played the ingenuous maid, assuring me I could bring up any subject I wished. I told her that I didn't know which ones. Karl laughed and wondered whether I wanted him to wait outside. Ginny was clever, witty and lovely today. When I said "well, I'll just take a chance and select at random," Ginny said straight-faced that if I ask the right question I'd get a free refrigerator.

Although I really wanted them to discuss sex, I thought I'd better start with a safer topic. I asked Ginny how she now felt about Karl's family; does she still feel that he is ashamed of her and doesn't want to introduce her to them? They talked about that very briefly, and I wonder in retrospect whether they didn't deliberately gloss over the subject. They then moved on to Ginny's feelings about her sister's engagement and then to Karl's bad relationship with one of their friends, Steve. When Karl started to explain his quarrel with Steve, I had to confess that I already knew about it; it must have been a strange experience for Karl to have seen me only twice and yet realize how very well I know him. I feel close to Karl and like him. I have to dig my spurs into myself to jar me out of the blind matchmaker role. My work with Ginny doesn't hinge on their getting married; what does matter is the quality of their relationship. Once experienced, a deep and honest intimacy will be with each of them forever, even if they were never to see one another again. I believe, with the faith of a convert, that this encounter may enrich future, yet unmet loves.

Then Ginny stated, almost in passing, that as a matter of fact she had talked to Karl just last night about sex. I was astounded, although I tried not to show it. Specifically, she had told him that she "needs some help" in getting full satisfaction. Subsequently she lay awake for two or three hours trembling, fearing she'd really upset Karl, and then had the courage to ask him how he felt (he had been awake too, worrying about other things). He answered that he hadn't been at all upset by that. Ginny's fear was that they had felt so close all day and that somehow she was "spoiling" things by bringing up a problem, as though it would mar their perfect day. I wanted Karl to let her know that the contrary was true. It was exactly the reverse: when she brings up a "problem" she doesn't distance him, but draws him closer. Karl agreed with me and I told him that I wished he would even say it again. And I gradually told him quite explicitly what Ginny had already suggested, which is almost their last remaining secret—that Ginny's worst time of day is the night, and it is her fear of what happens after she turns off the light that so terrorizes her days. Once that was made very explicit, and once Karl really knew it, I felt it was one of the most powerful therapeutic acts I've ever taken. I repeated myself a couple of times so that he would fully understand. I reiterated to Ginny that she can now share her anxieties with Karl and that the night panic doesn't have to happen again.

We moved from there to my asking Karl whether the reverse was ever true—whether he ever worried about Ginny's criticizing him or judging him, and he said he never did. So I pressed harder by asking, well, does he care whether she cares about him, and he said, that's true, he does care very much. And then we got into some interesting material where he admitted that he deliberately doesn't allow himself to think about that because then he doesn't have to worry about losing something, or losing Ginny. I told him he pays a very dear price for his feigned indifference and ostensible lack of worry—the price is distance, distance from others and from his love for others. He agreed with me, adding that that's why last night was such an unusual experience for him; today he could hardly wait to get home and felt so good about talking to Ginny. I imagined out loud that this whole business must have a long history. (I said that, I think, to help him start thinking about his past in preparation for his own therapy.) We ended up by apportioning our last three sessions. Ginny wants Karl to come again next week and perhaps the week after. She first said that she wanted at least a couple of sessions for herself, but now she says that she wants only the last one alone. She realizes, as do I, that the joint sessions are tremendously important.

May 31

GINNY

LAST SESSION was the most traumatic of the three. I was bringing in things to please you—the fact that Karl and I had been talking more openly. But you acted like we were two smug liars (not so strong). Of course, I was sitting on a powder keg and when you went fishing for new material, wondering what important topics had not been covered, I knew the end of my silence was near. The night before in a surge of warmth and truth toward Karl, I had started to broach the subject of my sex problems. As soon as I did, I realized I had kicked my foot in my mouth. We were just getting close, and before we could relish it very long, I gave us a problem that's so large and crucial, and one, as you always reiterated, which wasn't a good place to start with. "Start with small things like gasoline money," you'd say, but we were too close to bring up bridge tolls and stuff. Anyway, we talked about sex for awhile that night and after that, when we both tried to go to sleep I had my usual excruciating time. Unwilling to toss and ulcerate till dawn I asked Karl what he thought of what I had said. And he told me he was glad it had been talked about and we would go on from there.

So the following day when you asked what's new, was I nervous! I sat there nearly fainting, telling you nothing was wrong. Then you brought up Karl's reluctance to confirm me with his parents. This was not as crucial—I didn't care whether or not you brought it up because Karl not only withholds me from his parents, he withholds himself from them. I think he will have to come home to his parents first before he can take me home with him. But I think you were fishing for just how far you could go into sacred topics.

I brought up sex, feeling so ridiculous and matronly, as though I were middle aged with a tea cup and a topic sentence. I didn't want to waste the session, being deadpan. I can't remember too much of what we said, except that I said a lot, and wished I could have amnesty and have nothing held against me afterward.

By opening the subject, I have left myself open to the most wonderful hopes and worst punishments. Everyday is like therapy now. And change is the goal. I don't think that's ever been my goal before. I no longer need you to play Karl's part, he plays it all the time now, and I try to tell him things. The secrets and intrigues we had are all coming out and I don't know what's taking its place. I'm making contact with gut reactions. Karl playing himself is more forceful than you playing him. Only because there are consequences.

I tried to reassure Karl after session that every night I don't lie there at the edge of destruction. I wish we had started this long ago. Now that there is such a strong undertow.

I'm coming face to face with my own resistance.

May 31

KARL

I DON'T have any comments on the session itself. All this week and the week before I have been preoccupied with my article and since I have been working well, I haven't been anxious for too much psychological trauma which might prevent me from continuing. I have, however, tried to bring out Ginny and we have gotten some things said, but this has been a little one-sided since I always make sure that I am well in control of myself before saying anything to her about myself. I am talking around my core; I am not telling her my deepest, awfulest fears and compulsions possibly because I don't quite face them myself, but also because it would be an unburdening that would leave me helpless before her and I'm not sure I want that. Isn't that, I wonder, something to be saved for someone else? On the other hand I have, like Ginny, trouble experiencing immediate sensations, particularly physical ones, without feeling ironic about myself and the situation, so that I don't know whether the problem is mine or whether she is the wrong one, and that with another woman the problem of feeling would not present itself so strongly.

June 7

DR. YALOM

THIS WILL probably be the last time I see Karl, the last two sessions having been promised to Ginny alone. This hour was in many ways a downer compared to last week and I was somewhat disappointed by the suspense, caution, tenseness, and distance in the session. Ginny was obviously anxious: her legs were crossed tightly and her little foot was shaking back and forth. Karl gave an appearance of being extremely relaxed. He did something that I have never seen

195

anyone do in my office, which was to take off his heavy boots and sit there in his socks. Ginny was taken aback, asked what he was doing and said she wished he would at least have worn darned socks, as one had a hole in it. I felt that somehow or other this was a comment by Karl on his and my parity, which was important for him in maintaining his place in the relationship with the three of us. (And thus I said nothing.)

Grindingly, laboriously, we finally unearthed an issue. Last night while watching election returns, Ginny had fallen asleep and Karl barked at her, saying she would never change. This told by Ginny. When Karl told the story it then turned out that what he meant by "you'll never change" was that he had some sexual plans for that evening. He was waiting for Ginny to be more lively and assertive and instead she fell asleep. It was very disturbing for me to realize that Ginny had neglected to mention the sexual component of the story; it made me shudder to think of what an unreliable reporter of events she may have been in the past and how much time we may have spent dealing with issues which were the purest of gossamer in substance.

At any rate it became clear that Ginny felt censured by Karl; she was the judged and he was the judger. The election night incident represented in microcosm so much that goes on between the two of them. I told Ginny, for example, that she has a tremendous amount of evidence which demonstrates how much she has changed, even over the past few weeks; how then can she accept his definition of her as a person who doesn't change? That was a superb try on my part but utterly without impact.

Another attempt was to contrast their different perceptions of change. Karl wants some outward behavioral sign, whereas Ginny has made many changes in the way she feels about him, although it may not get translated into behavior. I then suggested to Karl that perhaps he ought to try to enter into Ginny's experiential world in order to perceive her sense of change. That fine suggestion was scarcely acknowledged.

The next thing I did, which usually gets results when something is really screwy in the atmosphere, was to comment on how strained I thought everything was today. Karl said that he had been feeling weird and it had something to do with his group therapy meeting. From there he soon moved into the admission that he does seem to have a need to be dominant to people and to encounter new people around the issue of dominance. If he can be dominant to others, he then loses interest in them and writes them off. But those people who present a challenge are the ones whose opinions concern him, perhaps even unduly. I tried to make him see how different it is for Ginny, who approaches individuals from an opposite set. In fact, Ginny looks, she said, for individuals who can dominate her. She likes to idolize and idealize individuals.

I tried to reinforce some of the things that we did last week to consolidate our gains. I reminded them that the old taboos are dead, that we had new, enlightened rules and encouraged them to continue taking gentle risks with one another. Apparently they had an extremely good day on Sunday when they went out to dinner because Ginny was somehow able to make it clear to Karl that she wanted to go out to dinner; they've done some talking and she's been feeling closer to him than ever before. All in all, however, I found myself not entirely satisfied with Ginny. I wanted her to perform better and I felt like a frowning parent disapproving of my child's timidity. She knows better, she can do better. "Stand up and speak out!"

Karl began the hour, incidentally, as he had the previous one, by asking me if he could get a cup of coffee, which I thought was in the same general ballpark as taking off his boots. While he was getting the coffee, Ginny mentioned that she wished we had started this so much sooner, things seemed to be moving so much more quickly now. She's right, of course, but forgets that they weren't ready for it when I urged her to bring Karl in months ago. Sometimes I wonder why I ever see a patient individually without at some point seeing the next closest person. I'm not sure, however, how much more work we could do on a long-term basis; maybe just a few sessions like this and then going back to the individual setting might be the best thing for them.

June 7

GINNY

I FOUND it difficult to talk. I wanted to keep "THE THING IN THE NIGHT" private. We weren't very explicit and I was pretty uncomfortable because everything that happens now has im-

197

mediate repercussions. Was it me who finally brought up the subject? Talking about the incident of my falling asleep the night before, you got to hear Karl's version and mine, and we both got to hear each other's. I became confused. You thought I was talking about the election returns when I was talking about sex. I thought that was obvious, and didn't need more translation. I guess I don't give enough strength to my voice and words, and allow them to settle about me like vapor.

Karl is a night person able to undergo hours of television and then expect a lively time about twelve-thirty, but grass and TV always leave me sleeping after an animated short while. In the early morning, however, I'm fine, refreshed, and Karl is like a seventh-month fetus, not ready to face the world, snarling not talking. My sleeping habit to him is a real character flaw; his goes unnoticed by himself.

You concluded that Karl thought I was unchanging. I guess you were disappointed when I agreed with him, thus confirming his verdict. I believe I am unchanging in the sense that, unlike him, I've never gone after something just to succeed; sometimes it happens naturally or miraculously. However, I do sprout new leaves. And hopes, which is my innocent, flimsy version of an ego. In session I changed, and at home with Karl my range of emotions and daring were greater. But I still allowed myself to be led by the rope in session, and only tentatively took the initiative.

Karl talked a lot about how he's limited his friendships because dominance has always been so crucial to him. And you said that maybe I wasn't enough of a challenge for him and that's why he resented and dismissed me so often. I thought you did this to show his weaknesses as well as mine. And each one of your sentences was like a free handout to me, a giveaway topic sentence. You wanted me to leap in; you sounded the bugle call.

There's a lot I wanted to say last session. I felt constrained and embarrassed. To me Karl is giving two messages—an opening of the door, a patience, a freedom, an understanding, but on the other hand he envisages certain progress, certain clarity of expression, healthy steps. Mirror imaging his own hopes. He expects these now from me immediately, as though they can be delivered like milk. Especially in sex; he wants me to strip away all the negative layers of fears and "I can't's". An instant overnight evolution. He's saying, "I want your freedom and I want it now." He's less patient than you, less ready to hold a microscope over my new small accomplishments.

I am amazed how Karl grows. Even his weaknesses seem to enlarge him. He has so many resources within himself. It is as if he has the possibility of becoming so many people, and not remaining entrenched in his own personality.

June 7

KARL

I JUST READ over what I wrote for you last week and it seemed like it was written by someone else. I don't know quite what I was thinking of I feel now that I have to have some thoughts and I just don't. It was easy enough for me in the early sessions, when I didn't feel so personally concerned, to sit back afterward and think about what went on, but the last two, after which I felt completely drained, have been something I have had to recover from. During the sessions I wasn't observing, which is what I am used to doing, and now, although I remember what we talked about and remember feeling that my life and my problems seemed very clear to me, that feeling is gone now. I cannot say so succinctly now what I said then, and the feeling of being intimate with you and Ginny and myself is now much less intense. Ginny and I have talked and I have tried to give to her, to tell her what my stomach squeezes tight in a last effort to keep hidden. It has all been very disturbing to me. I haven't written one word on my article since last Tuesday because when I sit down to write I find I have lost confidence in what I am writing and that then makes me doubt myself even more and makes it even harder to write anything. Then I tear myself away from my desk and do what I can to calm myself down. When I get calm, which usually takes until evening, I also feel empty because I don't think I have done

anything worthwhile. Another day of my life is gone and I have
done nothing but exhaust my nerves. Ginny is no help to me during
times like that and I don't know who would be. My old values, bad
and confining as they were, are disintegrating and I don't know quite
what to replace them with. When I write, this translates into my
not being able to find an appropriate point of view and I want to
write something that reflects more than confusion. I can understand
why patients build up a dependence on the therapist, and I don't
want that and I think it tends to make me reticent about the
sessions themselves. I think deep down my fear is that none of this
is going to work. That's my problem to deal with, but right now,
feeling another day of inactivity coming on me, I'm ending up
afraid.

June 14

DR. YALOM

THE next-to-the-last interview. It started off badly. Ginny knocked
on the door, I told her to come in, it was already fifteen minutes after
the hour. I looked absolutely astonished because I had totally forgotten our appointment, being preoccupied with some pressing writing. I don't think this related to Ginny because, in fact, I had already
done the same thing with two other patients this week. I am under
a great deal of pressure before getting away this summer to finish a
chapter for a book and prepare a talk for a large annual conven-
tion this Saturday. So it took me a minute or two to get oriented and
I mumbled something to Ginny about my secretary not being here
today, which was true, and that I had forgotten to keep track of the
time.

Then we started off and the opening five minutes were enough to
really throw me into despair. Jesus, it was the same old Ginny.
Things were tense and tight, she talked about wishing Karl were
here so he could make things go. She talked about her feelings of lifelessness and her long sieges of fantasy. She talked about phasing out

of the interview, as she has so often in the past. She went off into a long business about the fact that she can't have an orgasm with Karl and that she feels that this is going to be the deciding and fatal factor for the two of them.

I was beginning to sink into a hopeless pit. Why is everything so goddamned complicated? Why can't there ever be a happy ending? Why can't she take what she's gotten from me, keep it and own it and make it a part of her? I was so stunned that I acted like an automaton whose behavior was programmed from one of our sessions of six months ago. I questioned her exclusive fixation on the sexual issue. There obviously were many other important things going on between her and Karl. It sounded peculiar to me for her to consider the whole relationship as revolving around the axis of the orgasm. Surely she was not going to continue to measure her whole worth in terms of orgasmic units. I told her that if sex were really the problem, we could do something about that; she could go to a sex counselor, to people who specialize in the Masters and Johnson technique. I made many old-time unhelpful comments like this, sensing all the while a kind of willfulness in her plunging regression.

About that time I suddenly came to my senses and began to use my head; and it all became very clear to me. I had to understand what she was doing in the terms of "termination," which was now looming very large. I reminded her that although we've planned a meeting in the fall, it would just be a single hour, and we must really consider this to be our next-to-the-last session. Then I grew absolutely convinced that the reason she was feeling lifeless was to prevent herself from feeling strong emotions about our impending separation. I bit into that interpretation and hung on like a bulldog the rest of the hour, and am convinced that it was the right thing to do. I was so clever trying all the cute little stunts I could think of to help her remove herself just a bit from the situation but still be able to express her feelings about me and ending therapy. When she said she was saving up her emotions for next week, I asked if she could say today what she would say then. I wondered if she could foresee the contents of the letter she would write me this summer. I wondered if she could tell me what she would be feeling at this very moment, if her lifelessness weren't so consuming today. Gradually things began to come out—she would miss me. She was so jealous in the first session when I paid a lot of attention to Karl and she was very upset when Karl asked if he could come back next time, knowing she would have to share me with him, though it worked out for the best, she admitted. She thought I was so great in the way I dealt with Karl and she had so much admiration for me and so great a feeling of trust for me. She would miss me. There would be a big void in her life. She's been seeing me privately for almost two years and was in group therapy with me for a year and a half before that. Then she said that if she weren't really lifeless and had to talk about her feelings, she would have to cry a great deal and face very deep emotions and then what would she do next week? I told her at least half a dozen times I was absolutely convinced her lifelessness was there today to prevent her from experiencing and expressing what she was feeling. I wondered if she would be embarrassed to communicate to me some of her positive thoughts about me. She said that she would miss me and I told her I would miss her too. She said that she has seen people in group therapy as she is now, just waiting for the right question. I asked her what the right question would be and when she said, "What are your feelings about Dr. Y?" I repeated her words. She began to cry, and admitted that she was indeed experiencing some very powerful feelings which she doesn't usually allow herself to feel; they were good kinds of feelings and she doesn't know why she won't let them out. She said that it's masochistic because she knows it would be good for her to share these emotions with me. She would miss my sense of humor—it was different from Karl's.

I wondered if my keeping her waiting at the beginning of the hour didn't contribute to the lifelessness. She denied this but I'm not totally convinced. She said that she didn't mind my being late because, in a sense, she could spend a little more time in my environment. However, at the beginning of the session when I asked her how she felt about stopping, she said, "How much longer could you go on with me?" As if she were someone so disgusting that I could not continue seeing her. I couldn't get her to elaborate on that self-deprecating question but I'm sure that intermingled with all the positive feelings are also some negative ones, such as anger at my leaving; and her lifelessness in part reflects a punishment. I tried to get into this with her by commenting that even though she wasn't experiencing any conscious annoyance with me for stopping, her actions were expressing it for her. For example, she feels she's not doing very good write-ups for me and that she's generally regressing, which obviously disappoints me, since I would be so greatly pleased at any sign of continued progress in herself and with Karl.

She pointed out a number of ways that the joint sessions have been helpful, primarily in facilitating communication between her and Karl to an extent that would have been unthinkable before my sessions with them. She went so far as to aver that the sessions wouldn't be totally wasted even if Karl should decide to leave her —they're something she can own and carry into other situations.

She looked forward almost with glee to writing me long letters but I think that's a way of avoiding termination; expressing love long-distance probably seems easier. I didn't reveal too much of my feelings toward her today except to say I would miss her, and I reflected on the cruelty of psychotherapy which prizes caring, yet severs it mechanically. She seemed very moved at the end of the interview and I think the lifelessness was gone. She did something she's never done before—she held out her hand to me, although reluctantly. I shook her hand and touched her shoulder as she was leaving the office. How obscene it is that I had forgotten she would be here today. When I am with her she fills my life so much; it's amazing to me that I put her out of my mind at other times during the week. I guess compartmentalization like this is necessary for survival in this crazy business of titrated love.

June 14

GINNY

ON THE BUS home I had plenty of time to steep in my own thoughts and juices. You might be right that this lifeless show-and-tell I brought you is a shield against having to experience the end of therapy with you. I can't bear to think about it. Maybe that's why the next-to-last week I bring you a résumé of troubles and undone things. To show you I can't graduate from you.

You said that if I allowed my feeling to flow, therapy would really be over. I'd know it. I can't bear not to see you any more. You kept asking me if I were angry about the rigged setup of therapy where you get so close and dependent and then cut off. Well, of course, I'm angry and the way I show it is my old pattern—hurt myself, drain and dull myself, so you know I am hurting, and so you end by feeling bad.

In the brief time when you almost succeeded in making me give something, feelings, tears, I was tingling all over, and still I couldn't go all the way, which would be more than the recording inside myself, but to take a fling and spontaneously say what hurt, what I felt and give it to you. Through the walls I could hear someone else in therapy next door weeping constantly.

What I did today, I did to protect myself. You wanted me to say how I felt about finishing and I didn't really do that. I said I liked you. (Lamely.) But that's different from thinking about ending. You've always thought I was fragile. That's because I have so much damn packing around me. I hope like anything that we can get close next week, or else I'll feel so indebted to you, so like I've failed.

I've always trusted you. And you've been good to me. Maybe I wanted more and that's why I fought you so this year. (Passively, by feeling in myself I wasn't growing a lot of the time.) I felt like I was goading you to some forceful act toward me. To get rid of the hanger-on, the disappointer.

If you suddenly were to surprise me with some extra months of therapy, I'm not sure I would be too happy, in spite of all this moaning. Some of my deadness I think is a reaction against the trap of therapy, of having to come in here each week and tell you how much I care about you, about me, about Karl. And having to come to life just so I can hurt.

Last week you kept reiterating that you wanted me to tell you what I thought of you, not for your sake but for my own sake. But I think it really was for you. Then you could have felt we had accomplished something. Some time, maybe later in the summer when it has sunk in, I could tell you or write you. And with that easy promise, I glide away. I keep praying away in my head to do something heroic for you, not today but tomorrow, tomorrow.

June 21

DR. YALOM

THE LAST HOUR. I feel very shaky, very sad and very moved. My feelings toward Ginny are among the best kind of feelings I have ever had. I feel very close, very warm, very unselfish and very tender toward her. I feel I know her fully and wish only good things for her.

It was such a difficult hour today, but then it's been like that all week. I'm leaving for ten weeks in a couple of days and I've had to say goodbye to so many patients, so many people, that it's tarnished my saying it to Ginny. For example, today I had two groups that I said goodbye to. One is a group of psychiatric residents which will resume again in approximately three months, but in that group there were two women who will not continue because they are finishing their training and I had to say goodbye to them, and both of them felt very moved and so did I, though not to the extent that I feel with Ginny. But anyway, it's been a week of goodbyes and a week of my coming face to face with the specter of termination which I read about in the literature and tell my residents they're not handling very well. How do you "handle" something that dwarfs you?

What was I supposed to do with Ginny today? Have her go over and tell me again how marvelous it's been, or how much I've helped her get in touch with her feelings about Karl, or try to give her some guidelines about the future, or review her progress, or what? We were both tormented, I no less than she. Both of us kept looking at the clock. I ended actually a minute or two early because I felt we couldn't stand it any longer and I just didn't want to have to play out the ritual of staying together for the whole fifty minutes. I asked her what she was thinking. She asked me what I was thinking. She had to strain to produce thoughts. One of the first things she said was that she had been physically ill after the last hour with flu, and that it generally happens that way after a particularly bad hour. That caught me by surprise and forced me to review in my mind the last hour. She said that she had been so selfish, hadn't

205

given anything, had in fact phased out. I told her that I was surprised to hear that since I thought she had done so much. Talking about last week was good; one firm little ledge of "therapeutic work" that we could stand on during the hour today.

I asked what she wanted to be doing in five or ten years from now. We talked about having children. She asked how old I was when I first had a child and I told her I was twenty-four. I tried weakly to ask if Karl's not wanting children might even propel her into making a choice about their future together—the well-worn issue of whether Karl is the only one in the relationship who has choices, a theme so hoary and encrusted I felt somewhat ashamed to present it. It's never made any impact and God knows it's not going to be helpful now. She's never going to be an active chooser. However, she is so charming that she will always be chosen and that's important too, I guess.

I was obviously feeling very disorganized today. My office was in its customary state of disarray; in fact, it looked something like a junk shop with papers, books, briefcases strewn all over the floor. I am leaving in a few days, and still have a couple of articles to finish up. She asked me what they were about, and then offered jokingly to help me clean the office, and suggested that we didn't have to stay the whole time. I tried to correct any feeling she might have that I was covertly intimating I was too busy to see her, but she knew I wasn't saying that. I almost considered for a while accepting her offer of helping me clean up. That idea seemed fetching to me. I wonder why. I guess it would have been a way of allowing her to give me something. A way also of our doing something together other than this routinized psychotherapy, since that's what we call being together.

She lamented her customary style of gliding along on life. I implied that it might be helpful for her to be without a therapist now, to be on her own power without the propulsion of the weekly hour which allows her to glide along for the rest of the week. When I asked if she planned to go into therapy again, she mentioned bio-energetics. I winced visibly, whereupon she commented, "There you go, being gossipy again." Did she really forgive me for setting a time limit on therapy? After all, if I really cared for her, I would go on seeing her forever. Ginny didn't respond to that directly, but said that she realizes there are other people who need me more, although sometimes she has tried to hide her progress from me, perhaps as a punishment in retaliation for my ending therapy. She talked a good deal about next autumn, about writing me, about my knowing her address, about where I would be, about wanting to continue knowing me personally. I told her that she could write to me in France, that I would like to continue knowing her, but I also wanted her to know for sure that we were really at the end of her therapy. The letter writing and the single visit we would have in the fall would not diminish that fact. She said that she really did understand.

When I stopped the hour and said, "Well I guess the time has really come for us to say goodbye," we both of us remained frozen for a few seconds. She started to cry and said, "You are so wonderful to have done this for me." I didn't quite know what to say but the words that came out of my mouth were "I've gotten a great deal from this too, Ginny." And so I have. I went up to her while she was still sitting to take her hand and she put her arm around me and just hung to me for a minute and I put my hand in her hair and stroked her. I think that is the first time I've ever embraced a patient like that. It filled me with tears. And then she left the office, not a border-line character disorder, an inadequate personality, an obsessional psychoneurotic, a latent schizophrenic, or any of the other atrocities that we perpetrate daily. She left as Ginny and I will miss her.

June 21

GINNY

YOU TAKE my petty coping and calm, and play down all the detours that I take to get there. I admit I'm capable now of leading a normal life. In your office it seemed like I was trumping up problems. But sometimes my life seems very limited, without roots to real nourishment. I'm like a house plant firmly entrenched in a pot. Unless I am watered and moved, taken to the sun and away from it, I won't last. But even with some of my roots exposed, sticking out of the flower pot into the air, and even with the pot too small, I'm doing nicely. There is a chance I can go on like this without need of being transplanted.

Maybe living my life like I am now, posing small problems for myself, like the house and food, will give me some small encouragement. And Karl is a whole new ballgame.

I imagine psychiatry as being able to bridge the gap between the real self and the hibernating, dreamt self. I'm in a calm siege now holding out against my inside. I feel okay.

I wonder how mundane I can get before you give me an A for recovery. I don't want to be dynamited out of my warmed curled-up self. I prefer to lull myself into excited memory. Or so it seems.

Our problem together is still defining what is real. So much of what you do and I say in session, I frown at in retrospect. I suppose I had illusions of spilling out of my cleavage this last session with emotions and tears. I've seen too much theater. And maybe I am angry that I have not turned into a mental patient under your guidance, and that I couldn't give you more of a fight.

And sometimes I think "what the hell"? I feel like dandelion fuzz, blowing in the breeze, not settling anywhere, yet. I feel ecstatic, even though that old chorus sings, "What do you have to be ecstatic about?" At least you are my friend, and I envision the day when I can pound on your door.

Doctor Yalom's Afterword

THE "FINAL" SESSION was not the last meeting with Ginny. Four months later, shortly before Ginny left California permanently, we talked again. It was a tense and melancholy meeting for me, not unlike seeing an old girlfriend and straining to recapture the once lovely, now withered mood. We didn't "do therapy" but chatted informally about the summer and the impending move.

She loved her summer job as a teacher of children in a child development project, and instead of writing dry observational research notes, apparently overwhelmed the research team with picturesque and poignant observations of the children. I chuckled as I imagined their faces reading her reports.

The dreaded calamity had occurred: Karl had decided to take a job in a city two thousand miles away. But he made sure to tell her in a number of ways that he wanted her to come with him. Ginny felt clearly that she had more than one choice—she could go with Karl, live with him, marry him, but if that didn't work out, she felt easy with the thought of making a life without him. She seemed less desperate, more confident. I no longer experienced her as lying on a taut sheet of anxiety.

Ginny moved away with Karl and passed out of my mind for several months until the day when I stuffed our reports into a briefcase, brought them home and asked my wife to read them. My wife's reaction persuaded me to consider the material for publication, and ten months after our final interview I phoned Ginny to discuss it with her. Though she had reservations, she was willing for our venture to be published (so long as she could protect her anonymity) and we each agreed to edit our parts, to write a foreword and afterword, and to share royalties equally. Over the phone I detected none of the old, desperate stagnation so typical of Ginny early in her treatment. She sounded (as, of course, I wanted her to sound) active and optimistic. She had made some new close friends and was actively writing. She had sold her first piece of writing for three hundred dollars, an uncanny event since it precisely fulfilled a fantasy she had described to me at the beginning of therapy. Things with Karl still sounded unsettled, but it was clear that the rules of the relationship had been changed: Ginny appeared more powerful and more resourceful.

A few days later I received a long letter from her, which I quote in part:

Dear Dr. Yalom:

. . . I don't know how I feel. I go from hot flashes to pushing it out of my mind, to concentrating on the money factor which I certainly could use. I wish my part were better. In looking back, I only spent a few minutes on the write ups some times. However, that's just me. I am trying to finish my novel now—and I write five pages a day, which sounds great except that it takes me about fifteen minutes a day to write five pages. I've always written fast. I write by the rhythm method— just sounds and rhymes, no intellectual thoughts, no thinking. It all seems to be ordained, this spontaneous backlog of words. Mine are so sloppy—you must be thinking this was subconscious on my part to throw you off the track from publishing them. I wish my life were different now so I could feel those write ups were distant memories, and I have now gone to bigger and better things and emotions. I felt stuck so much of the time in therapy—the only time I ever got my pinions was when I cried. I felt like I had taken my giant steps when we first knew each other, and that somehow I've been taking little tied Japanese steps back ever since, except for a few melodramatic psychodramas when I could be the emotional character I've always wanted to be. This is all an exaggeration, of course. I know some wonderful things hap- pened—the best—our friendship. If you think the write ups will have some value, I trust you.

Let me tell you a little about my life here.

. . . X is very much like Palo Alto without its lushness or money. The University is pre-sixties. The student body is so calm—if you gave them a brick, unlike at Berkeley, they would just begin to make a barbeque pit with it, never think of smashing a window. We live in an old house with a backyard that looks like where old fishing rods come to die—it is filled with living and dead bamboo.

. . . I took a big job as a freelance writer, and recently sold a short story for $300. I've also done some articles for a magazine. . . . I recently attended a woman's consciousness raising group and wrote some personal observations about it which will be published. I will send it to you when it comes out. It's lucky they didn't ask for each woman to come forth with her story. I would have to call mine "Ginny and the Gasoline Money."

. . . Karl's and my relationship has not changed much. We are still comfortable with each other, and sometimes loving. We've had our quota of late night dramas where I've slipped back into the terrible fear. I'm still in that nightly labyrinth. We are just ourselves, which is not too emotional but friendly. I speak out now. A while ago Karl told me that I had no goals or ends. I gave us three months to try and evaluate our relationship . . . the longer I stay here the closer Karl and I become, but I have no direction and our future seems like a sentence that can either be kept or edited out.

. . . I am feeling fine. Most of the time I'm happy—though my mind can go either way. When I force myself to write, for however short a time, I'm happy. I waited so long to write to you because I have always imagined myself as on a brink and I'm waiting for the story to send you that you want to hear.

. . . Karl, in one of our fights and resulting deadly silences, said—"Oh, I was just thinking of Dr. Yalom wishing he were here." We both send our love. Your friend,

Ginny

Then silence. I took up my role with the other Ginnys in my life participating in the dramas which unfolded on the revolving stage of my office. No! How pretentious! And how untrue! I know how much of myself I give to each of my patients and the truth is I gave more to Ginny. More of what? What is it that I gave more of? Interpretations? Clarifications? Support? Guidance? No, something on the other side of technique. My heart went out to Ginny. She moved me. Her life was precious to me. I looked forward to seeing her. She was starving but very rich. She gave me a great deal.

Some fourteen months after the "final session" she visited California and we met twice. First, a work-social meeting with my wife. Ginny arrived, accompanied by her best friend. Ginny wanted us to meet but had cautioned me before to say nothing that would betray that we were writing a book together. That made for some awkwardness. The friend, a dark-haired charmer, stayed a few minutes. When she left it was just Ginny, my wife, and me. We discussed the manuscript and chatted over sherry, tea and some goddamn homemade cookies. Not knowing what I wanted, I knew what I didn't want—small talk and the intrusion of others.

I abhor the professional-social marshland. We try to appear at ease but are not. Ginny shows her social manners. She acts, she tries to amuse my wife, but we both know she is barely paddling ahead of a tidal wave of self-consciousness. We are conspirators, we participate in the social charade and pretend we do not. My wife calls me Irv, Ginny cannot mouth the word and I continue orbiting as Dr. Yalom. I do not give her explicit first name instructions under the spell of some murky rationalization that she needs to keep me in professional orbit for use at some future time. Even more bizarre is my recoil at my wife's familiarity with me in front of Ginny. I forget, what was it I was planning to do for Ginny? Oh yes, "to aid reality testing so that she would work through her positive transference."

A few days later Ginny and I talked in the snug, unambiguous comfort of my office. There, at least, each of us "knows our place." We analyzed our feelings at the social meeting. Ginny's friend so lauded me for my warmth and ease (so much for her perceptivity!) that Ginny pummeled herself for not having taken more advantage of her time with me. One interesting thing occurred before we started. She presented herself to my new secretary who asked, "Are you a patient?" Ginny replied quickly, "No, I'm a friend." That felt good to both of us.

My wife was waiting to talk to Ginny about some sentences in the manuscript and twice during our talk knocked on the door. The first time I said that we'd be five more minutes. But we talked for much longer, and my wife, growing impatient because she had another appointment, knocked again. This time Ginny preempted me and, to my amazement, said almost sharply, "just a few more minutes." When the door closed she burst into tears, real tears, as the present flooded in: "I just realized I really have only a few more minutes. It's not that your wife has you all the time but this time is really precious to me." She cried for both of us, for the time we would never have again, for joy at having, finally, "spoken out" and (alas) from sadness at not having spoken up more in her life. (We were both saddened by the reappearance of that pleasure-stripping imp who berated her, even in the midst of success, for not having succeeded even more.)

A short time after she returned home Ginny sent me a letter with dramatic news:

. . . When I got home again Karl and I were kind of strangers again. . . . He sort of ignored me, and I felt like a child ignored by a father. Karl could deprive me of things—going swimming, doing this, doing that. If he didn't want to do it, we just didn't go. Finally I confronted Karl and said that we weren't getting along at all. He said "I know. I want out.". I didn't protest this time, and by the next day Karl had already moved out. (Two days ago). . . . No one blames the other and maybe we didn't have any future. It's now the second day and I have a hollow stomach but my mind is much better. I don't intend to fall apart. I just feel awfully sad and unbelieving. At first I thought I was going to go right back to California. But I would rather have my feet on the ground and try to live my life alone—independently so I'll have done it and don't ever have to be scared again. I'm going to stay here as long as I can. Karl says he was burned out with me. I believed it. I sensed it. . . . I want to get healthy and strong—I want to struggle out of this. I'm beginning to have insights. When my worst moments come, when I become desperate, I just have faith that it must pass and that you can't die from hurting. (A mucky line!) In crying, though it leads nowhere, at least it is something, and as you know, I'm partial to tears. If things get too bad here, I'll go to a doctor who can give me some Valium, but I'm a Christian Scientist when it comes to tranquilizers. Last night I slept O.K., and I woke up feeling sad but not really scared.

I know that I'll be able to make it here, and I'm going to start looking for a job. I know the next few weeks will be slow and hurting. I keep forgetting and remembering, not being able to believe that Karl won't be here again. We didn't part in anger, just sadness.

Though she hadn't asked for it, I crammed some gratuitous psychotherapy into an envelope and shot it back to her.

Dear Ginny:
A shock all right, but not without premonition on my part too. I feel badly for how badly you are feeling now and will feel for the next couple of months, but yet I don't feel unambivalently badly, and I can see by your letter that you don't either. I think the fact that Karl was able to do this and do it apparently so quickly means, to me, that he has been doing it in his head for a long period of time. I don't believe things like that can be done in one's head without the other person getting some sense of it which has resulted in a kind of global, dulled feeling for you, and which has restrained your growth over these months. All I can do to help (which I know you are not asking me to do) is just to remind you that what you are in the midst of will pass. After your shock and feelings of panic, I suspect a period of real grief at your loss and a feeling of hollowness or emptiness might set in. Perhaps even then some feelings of anger (God forbid), but the course of such things is always something around two to three to four months, and after that I think you will come out on the other side much stronger than ever.

I am really impressed with the strength that you seem to be summoning now. If there is anything that I can do to help during this bad period, please let me know.

With the tunnel vision of a surgeon who is convinced that his operation was successful, regardless of the fate of the patient, I was convinced that her letter was full of strength. The break with Karl did not token a failure: therapeutic success is not synonymous with her making it with Karl (though I had, myself, slipped into that error during our first joint sessions.) Furthermore, Ginny had played some part in the final break, though not as active a part as she would have liked. It is quite common that, when one member of a pair changes and the other does not, the balance of their relationship is so altered that they cannot stay together; possibly Ginny outgrew Karl, or at least now realized that, because of Karl's judgmentalism, the relationship is stunting for her; possibly only now can she really envision living without Karl and permit him to leave her. After all, he often intimated that he wanted out but since he believed that she would disintegrate, he was bound to her by guilt, the most unsatisfactory cement for a union. Perhaps now Karl recognized her increased strength. Perhaps now they were both liberated and could act with freedom in their best interests.

My optimism was confirmed. I learned from phone conversations over the next four months that she reacted marvelously well. She mourned her loss, licked her wounds and then opened her door and walked out into the world. She sought out friends; she got a full-time job as a writer for a literary foundation and continued to freelance; she dated, soon selected a man and gradually developed a deep and tender relationship with him. She feels content and most comfortable with him, partly because of his characteristics—he is nonjudgmental, gentle and solicitous—and, I like to think, partly because of her new strengths and her increased ability to communicate, to trust and to love.

* * *

The closest this book came to not being published occurred when I asked a colleague, a devout Freudian analyst whom I much respect, to read the manuscript. After reading the first thirty pages, he commented that "this is what Wilhelm Reich used to call the 'chaotic situation,' where the therapist says to the patient whatever happens to spring to mind." Happily, several favorable readings by other colleagues provided sufficient reassurance to permit me to publish the book and to refrain from altering the text. Still, as I reread the manuscript there is an appearance of capriciousness in my actions, which conceals the fact that the entire course of therapy took place within the framework of a generous but rigorous conceptual system. In the following pages I shall describe that system and discuss the therapeutic principles which guided my behavior.

Recall, first, the state of affairs at the beginning of our individual work together. Ginny chugged into individual therapy leaving behind a wake of discouraged and defeated therapists; there were lessons to be learned, errors to be avoided. She had frustrated two highly competent analytically oriented psychotherapists who had endeavored to foster insight, to clarify the past, to modify the growth-stunting relationship with her parents, to interpret her dreams, to appreciate and diminish the influence of her unconscious on her waking life. A bioenergeticist had attempted unsuccessfully to reach and to change her via her body musculature; he had suggested muscle relaxation, new methods of breathing and tension relief via vomiting. She had met and outmaneuvered some of the best encounter group leaders who had not hesitated to use the very latest confrontational methods: nonstop marathon groups lasting twenty-four–forty-eight hours designed to erode resistance by sheer physical fatigue, nude groups to encourage total self-disclosure, psychodrama complete with mood music and dramatic stage lighting to enable her to do in the group what she never dared to do in life, "psychological karate" to help her reach and express her anger by a variety of rage-provoking techniques including physical assault, and vaginal massage with an electric vibrator to overcome sexual unease and to achieve vaginal orgasm.

She had staunchly resisted my best efforts and those of my co-therapists in group therapy for a year and a half, and we wearily decided that it made little sense to continue. Throughout this time, however, her strong positive feelings for me and her faith in my ability to help her never faltered. To be sure, this positive transference had, thus far, been more a hindrance that a boon to Ginny's therapy.

To explicate this last point let me make the distinction between primary benefits and secondary gratifications in psychotherapy. Patients seek therapy for some relief of suffering; this relief (and often the necessary concomitant personality change) constitutes the primary benefit—the raison d'être of psychotherapy. Not infrequently, however, the patient derives some strong gratification from the actual process of being in therapy; he may enjoy the unceasing, unending solicitude, the rapt attention paid to his every thought, the reassuring presence of the omniscient, protecting therapist, the state of suspended animation when no important decision need be made. Not infrequently the secondary gratifications may be so great that the wish to remain in therapy becomes greater than the wish to be cured.

Such was the state of affairs in Ginny's therapy. She attended the group not to grow but to be with me, she spoke not to work on problems but to gain my approval. As we learn from her therapy notes, she was not part of the group but part of the audience and cheered me on as I forged to the rescue of other stricken patients. Ofttimes the co-therapists and the other members observed that Ginny appeared to stay sick for me; to get well meant to say goodbye. And so she remained suspended in a great selfless wasteland, not so well as to lose me, not so sick as to drive me away in frustration.

How to turn this transference to therapeutic account? Surely there must be a way to harness Ginny's unswerving and, to some extent, irrational faith in me in the service of her own growth. And, since Ginny had moved to another city, how to do it with structural limitations that made it impossible for us to meet more than once weekly?

My overall plan was to orient therapy almost entirely around the axis of our relationship. I hoped to fix our gaze, insomuch as was humanly possible, on what occurred between Ginny and me in the immediate present. Our temporal-spatial territory was to be the here and now, and I planned to discourage any excursions away from this focus. We would interact intensively, analyze our interaction and repeat the sequence for as long as we were together. Simple enough, but how would this lead to therapeutic change? My rationale for this stance derives from Interpersonal Theory.

Briefly put, the theory of interpersonal relationships posits that all psychological disorders (which are not caused by some physical insult to the brain) stem from disturbances in interpersonal relationships. People may seek help from a psychotherapist for a variety of reasons (depression, phobia, anxiety, shyness, impotence, etc.), but underlying these reasons and common to all is an inability to establish satisfying and enduring relationships with other people. These relationship difficulties have their origins far back in the past in the earliest relationships with parents. Once established, disturbed methods of relating to others advance forward to color subsequent relationships with siblings, playmates, teachers, chums, lovers,

spouses and children. Psychiatry, then, becomes the study of interpersonal relationships; psychotherapy, the correction of distorted
interpersonal relationships; and therapeutic cure, the ability to relate
appropriately to others rather than on the basis of some pressing, unconscious personal needs. Although the origins of maladaptive behavioral patterns lay in the past, the correction of distortions can
occur only in the present and nowhere better than in the most immediately present relationship—that between patient and therapist.

One additional basic assumption is necessary to help us understand how the therapist-patient relationship can alter maladaptive
interpersonal patterns. The therapist assumes that the patient, provided that the atmosphere is a trusting and unstructured one, will
soon display in his relationship with the therapist many of his major
interpersonal difficulties. If he is arrogant, vain, self-effacing, deeply
suspicious, seductive, exploitative, alienated, frightened of closeness,
contemptuous or any of the infinite number of disturbed ways one
may be with others, then he will be that way as he relates to the
therapist. The therapy hour and therapist's stage become a social
microcosm. No need to take a history, no need to ask for descriptions
of interpersonal behavior; sooner or later the entire tragic behavioral
scroll is unrolled in the office before the eyes of both therapist and
patient.

Once the patient's interpersonal behavior is recapitulated on the
stage of the therapist's office, the therapist begins in a variety of ways
to help the patient observe himself. The here-and-now focus on the
therapist-patient relationship is thus a two-pronged one: first, there is
lived experience as the patient and the therapist interlock in a curious
paradoxical embrace, at once artificial and yet deeply authentic. Then
the therapist, as tactfully as possible, shifts the frame so that he and
the patient become observers of the very drama which they enact.
Thus there is a continual sequence of emotional enactment and reflection upon that enactment. Both steps are essential. Enactment
without reflection becomes simply another emotional experience, and
emotional experiences occur all our lives without resultant change.
On the other hand, reflection without emotion becomes a vacant
intellectual exercise; we all know patients, iatrogenic mummies, so
bound with insight and self-consciousness that spontaneous activity
becomes impossible.

Once the self-reflective loop is established and the patient is able to
witness his own behavior, the therapist helps to make him aware

of the consequences of his actions, both upon himself and upon others. This done, the real crunch of therapy begins: the patient must, sooner or later, ask himself, "Am I satisfied with this? Do I want to continue being this way?" Eventually every road in every form of therapy leads to this point of decision, and patient and therapist must linger there until the arrival of the energy-supplying core of the change process: *Will*. We make our puny attempts to hasten the development of *Will*. Generally we do battle with the forces of counter-will by attempting to demonstrate that the anticipated dangers of behaving differently are chimerical. Our efforts are, for the most part, however, effete and indirect; generally we perform rituals, make obeisances, or merely grit our teeth waiting for *Will* to emerge from the vast darkness in which it dwells.

The therapeutic edifice I have described has yet one more supporting beam, without which the whole structure would topple. The changes that occur in the inner sanctum of therapy must be generalizable. Therapy is a dress rehearsal; the patient must be able to transfer his new ways of behaving with the therapist to his outside world, to the people who really count in his life. If not, then he has not changed, he has merely learned how to exist graciously as a patient and will be in analysis interminably.

The flow chart I have just presented reeks of the experimental laboratory. Psychotherapy never has such steel-spectacled efficiency; it must be a deeply human experience—nothing vital can come of an inhuman mechanistic procedure. Nothing, then, so neat; therapy as it actually transpires is less contrived, less simplistic, more spontaneous than the flow chart suggests. The therapist does not always know what he is doing; at times confusion, even bedlam, reigns; the stages are not clearly demarcated and rarely sequential. Psychotherapy is a cyclotherapy, as therapist and patient together ascend a rickety, low gradient, spiral staircase.

Perhaps it would be appropriate now after reviewing these broad basic tenets of interpersonal psychotherapy to describe my initial impressions of Ginny's interpersonal pathology and how I hoped to help her. Ginny's basic interpersonal stance was one of self-effacement. There are, after all, many ways of approaching others: some people strive for dominance, others for acclaim or respect, others for freedom and escape. Ginny sought for one primary commodity from others—love, and at any cost.

Her basic interpersonal stance had pervasive ramifications for her inner life and her external behavior. It dictated what she would cultivate in herself and what she would suppress, what she feared and what she enjoyed, what filled her with pride and what with shame. She cultivated any trait which, in her appraisal, made her more lovable. So she nurtured the hostess parts of herself, her amusing chirping wit, her generosity, her selflessness. She suppressed traits which belied this idealized image of goodness: her rights were scarcely recognized, much less honored—they were sacrificed on the altar of self-effacement; rage, greed, self-assertiveness, independence and personal desire were all regarded as saboteurs to the regime of love—all were exiled to the remotest region of the mind. They surfaced only in impulsive, out-of-the-blue flashes or, heavily disguised, in fantasies and dreams.

More than anything else she feared loss of love and lived in terror of displeasing others: she responded to the threat of losing Karl's love with panic, not unlike the panic of a young child deprived of the care of individuals necessary for biological survival. Furthermore, she could never be loved enough. She could never stop pressing herself to be better, more selfless, more pleasing. She was not permitted personal pleasure; if she wrote well, or enjoyed sex, or simply basked in luxurious well-being, the other, flagellant self intervened in the form of an appropriate antagonist: guilt (and ensuing paralysis) for writing frivolously or briefly; ridicule or self-consciousness to stifle the approaching orgasm; charges of sloth to poison her well-being.

Ginny's interpersonal pathology was not subtle; when I first began working with her I was very aware of these patterns and their consequences for her growth. At the beginning of therapy I wanted to communicate my observations to her. I wanted very much to say two things: (1) Your frantic search for love is irrational; it is a frozen piece of ancient behavior transported into the present, and ill-suited for your adult life. Your panic at the threat of love-withdrawal, appropriate no doubt in earliest infancy, is similarly irrational; you are capable of survival without stifling nurturance. (2) Not only is your request irrational, but it is tragically self-defeating. You cannot possibly secure an adult love through childlike terror and self-effacement. To insure that their daughters obtained a husband, Chinese parents crippled them by binding their feet in early childhood. You do even greater violence to yourself. You suffocate the person you could become, you have condemned most of yourself to an early grave. You suffer from your daily travails and your small failures, but there is, underneath it all, an even greater suffering because you know what you have done to yourself.

But sentences cannot say these things. I was to say them many times and in many ways through the embrace of therapy.

I planned to get very close to Ginny, to encourage her to re-experience all these ancient, irrational needs in her relationship with me: her sense of helplessness and need for my nurturance, her fear that I would withdraw my love, her belief that she could keep me only by self-sacrifice and self-immolation, her conviction that I would abandon her were she to take adult-like strides. I hoped that we could periodically step back from our experience so that Ginny could not only understand her patterns of relating to me but also appreciate their limiting, crippling nature.

Once the relationship became potent and a self-reflective stance was established I hoped to demonstrate that she was capable of establishing a richer, more adult relationship with me. In effect, I hoped that Ginny would begin not only to grow increasingly dissatisfied with her present hierarchy of needs, not only in a wistful way to desire change, but to consider change as an actual possibility. I could forsee many tactics but my basic strategy would be to oppose, in any way possible, those forces which smothered her will. For example, Ginny rarely permitted her will to emerge because she feared that it was incandescent rage, that it would result in loss of control, massive retaliation and rejection. By reacting supportively and encouragingly to all glimmerings of self-assertive expression, I hoped to demonstrate to her the fanciful nature of her fears and help her progressively transform more of her wishes, through will, into action.

The plan to write and exchange reports appealed to me for many reasons. First, and most simply, it forced Ginny to write. She had been blocked for months. I knew I was on treacherous ground and had to walk carefully to stay on the side of Ginny the person who fulfilled herself deeply when she wrote. I had to avoid viewing and treasuring Ginny as an indispensable but inert receptacle containing a great and coveted gift.

The format had other, more subtle implications. Most important was that it reinforced the self-reflective loop in the here-and-now focus. There was no dearth of emotion between Ginny and me; in fact too often I found myself trying to shake free from the swirl of feelings that encircled us. Writing and reading the reports helped Ginny (and me, too) gain perspective, pull herself out of the eye of the storm, observe and understand her behavior with me.

The notes were also an exercise in self-disclosure for both of us. I hoped that Ginny in the peace of her solitude could give voice to some of the stifled parts of herself. I planned to reveal more of myself in the notes than my personal vanity and professional reserve permitted me to do in the sessions. I especially hoped that she, by appreciating my foibles, my doubts, my bewilderment and discouragement, would adjust her unrealistic over-evaluation of me. Her childlike looking-up-at-me-with-wonder gaze often made me feel helpless and lonely. I wanted her to know that. I wanted her to climb out of that antediluvian gully and look at me, touch me, talk to me face-to-face. If she could do that and if I could show her that I could accept, indeed, welcome the hidden parts of herself as, one by one, they poked their timid heads through the lattice work of her self-effacement, then I knew that I could help her grow.

To read the text that Ginny and I have written is an enriching experience for me; few psychotherapists have had the opportunity to review from a dual perspective the entire course of therapy in such exquisite detail. I am struck by many things. Let me begin with the obvious discrepancies in perspective between Ginny and me. Often she values one part of the hour, I another. I press home an interpretation with much determination and pride. To humor me and to hasten our move to more important areas she "accepts" the interpretation. To permit us to move to "work areas," I on the other hand humor her by granting her silent requests for advice, suggestions, exhortations, or admonitions. I value my thoughtful clarifications; with one masterful stroke I make sense out of a number of disparate, seemingly unrelated facts. She rarely ever acknowledges, much less values my labors, and instead seems to profit from my simple, human acts: I chuckle at her satire, I notice her clothes, I call her buxom, I tease her when we role play.

The analogy to Rosencrantz and Guildenstern is an important one for me. That the therapist is the protagonist in many, varied, simultaneous dramas *is* his ultimate terrible secret. Furthermore, despite all pretenses at total self-disclosure it is a secret that cannot be totally shared. It brings home with great vividness some of the paradoxes of psychotherapy. Our relationship is a deep and authentic one, yet it is antiseptically packaged: we meet for the prescribed fifty minutes, she receives computerized notices from the clinic business office. The same room, same chairs, same position. We mean much to one another, yet we are characters in a dress rehearsal. We care deeply for one another, yet we disappear when the hour is up, we will never meet again when our "work" is done.

I imply to Ginny that we strive for egalitarianism, yet the notes expose our essential apartheid. I write to a third person "Ginny," she to a second person "you." I do not, even in the safer recesses of the notes, reveal to Ginny what I expect her to reveal to me. Her visit to me is often the central part of her week; often she is one of several patients I see on a particular day. Usually I give her much of my presence but sometimes I cannot draw the curtains on earlier dramas with other patients. I expect her to take me into herself, to let me mean everything to her and yet, for the most part, I keep her compartmentalized in my mind. How can it be otherwise? To give everything to everyone every time is to leave nothing for yourself.

Despite the fact that the reports contain a vast number and variety of techniques, I have no sense that my therapy with Ginny was technique-oriented. Rather, the specific techniques were entirely expendable and employed in the service of the conceptual scheme I have presented. Though I shrink back at dissection, I shall attempt to demonstrate this by reviewing some of the techniques and discussing the rationale behind their use.

The major techniques I employed fall into three clusters: (a) interpretative (b) existential (c) activative (by which I mean exhortation, advice, confession and absolution, role playing couple therapy, behavioral modification, and assertive training).

Interpretation is a mode of illumination. Much of our behavior is controlled by forces which are not in awareness. One might in fact offer as a definition of mental illness that we are mentally ill to the extent to which we are guided by unconscious forces. Psychotherapy, as I practiced it with Ginny, strove to illuminate the darkness—to reclaim psychological territory from the unconscious by the floodlight of the intellect. The interpretative process was one stage of the effort to aid Ginny to assume active control of her life.

What kind of interpretations did I make? For what types of "insight" was I hoping? It is commonly assumed that interpretation, insight, and the unconscious refer only to the distant past. Indeed, to the very end of his life Freud held that successful therapy hinged on the complete reconstruction of early life events which shaped the mental apparatus and reside now in the unconscious. Yet, in my work with Ginny I did not attempt to excavate the past; on the contrary I assiduously avoided it and charged Ginny with "resistance" when she attempted to look backward.

I wished to help Ginny explore her unconscious (insofar as it shackled her) and I did not wish to explore the past. Is there a contradiction? I can best explain my stance by asking that you consider the unconscious as an abstraction consisting of two coordinates: a vertical, temporal coordinate and a horizontal, ahistoric cross-sectional coordinate. The vertical temporal coordinate extends backward into the past and forward into the future. The temporal historical, developmental coordinate is a familiar concept. Few will dispute that events from the distant past, long forgotten or repressed, shaped our personality structure and control much of our behavior. What is not so obvious is that we are also controlled by the "not yet"—by our projections into the future. The goals we have set for ourselves, the ways we wish to be regarded ultimately by others, the perspective cast on life by death, the longing we have to be remembered, all the diverse and symbolic forms assumed by our need for immortality— all may be out of awareness and all may profoundly influence our inner life and external behavior. We are as pulled by the magnet of the future as we are pushed by the deterministic thrust of the past.

But it was the horizontal ahistoric coordinate of the unconscious that was the particular target of my interpretative efforts. At any given moment in time there are layers upon layers of forces operating out of our awareness which influence our actions and feelings. For example, Ginny was influenced by the dictates of her idealized image, by the pride system which determined what aspects of herself she would value and what she would suppress, by her irrational need for love and her conviction that self-assertion was evil or dangerous. To be sure, one could argue that these unconscious ahistoric forces are shaped by past experiences. But that is not the point; temporal causality is an inessential frame of reference in the therapeutic endeavor. Archeological excavation, the search for the whence, the primordial cause—intriguing issues, but not synonymous with the therapeutic process. Not irrelevant either though. The intellectual chase often serves to maintain the therapist's interest and enthusiasm; it combines with the patient's dependency to form a therapeutic epoxy locking patient and therapist together long enough for the major instigator of change—the therapeutic relationship—to grind into movement. I enjoy the diggings also, but, if I can, I try to hold my curiosity in abeyance and to focus on the many-layered forces, conscious and unconscious, which, in the immediate present, shaped Ginny's thoughts, feelings and behavior.

Much of my interpretative work revolved around "transference" —Ginny's unrealistic relationship to me. Rather than discuss her reluctance to stand up for her rights or her inability to express anger in abstraction, I attempted to examine these difficulties as they were manifested in her dealings with me. Therefore, I tediously asked Ginny to express all of her feelings about me. My first task was to help her recognize feelings and later to express them. I had to rely on indirect evidence at first and deduce her feelings. She denies any strong feelings about me, yet regularly is sleepless or filled with panic the night before a session. She has a migraine headache immediately preceding or following the session, or vomits on the way to my office. When I cancel a session she has no reaction, yet she misses or arrives late for the next session or immediately lapses into a depression to punish me (through guilt) for my inconsiderateness. Often the richest vein to mine was her fantasy life: Karl leaves her, I take her away to a cabin in the woods, I care for her, feed her, send her my assistant for a sexual romp. Though she usually disowned them, these were her fantasies and, therefore, her wishes; I pursued them however I could. I confronted her continually about her behavior with me and encouraged her to take risks. Why could she not disagree with me? Ask me any questions? Dress attractively for me? Express her disappointment with me? Get angry? Tell me she cared about me? Later I will speak of the value of behaviorial change as a primary technique, here I employed behavior in the service of the interpretative approach. By encouraging her to dare do the things she dreaded, I hoped to make her aware of the opposing, frightening unconscious forces.

So I made interpretations—at first to assist her to retrieve the feelings that had been pushed into unawareness, then to suggest regular global patterns in her behavior, then to help her comprehend the unconscious assumptions which dictate these patterns.

But insight, even perfect illumination, is not enough. Change

225

requires an act of will. Earlier I described the elusive nature of will and suggested that, in one way or another, all techniques are ultimately aimed at rousing and strengthening will—the will to change, to grow, and, most important for Ginny, the will *to will*. Interpretative techniques are often the first steps toward the resuscitation of will. First we simply help the individual to be aware of the current which sweeps him along through life. Some unmoving object—a tree, a house, a silo, a therapist—is required to help the pilgrim patient know he is moving and not at his own volition. Once the existence of the current is appreciated then, through reason, the patient is helped to gauge the strength and the nature of the current. And so he becomes aware both of the absence of will and of the shape of the forces which have replaced it. Knowledge provides the first step toward mastery.

The existential and the activating techniques provide further steps in the development and maturation of will: existential techniques foment the germination process while activating techniques coax the tendril upward once it has broken through the earth. First consider the "existential" techniques. I encase the term in quotes and use it with trepidation because it has become abstruse and vulgarized. Like an old gavel or academic gown it is carted in to lend dignity to any occasion. Therefore, I shall be as precise as possible. By "existential" I refer to an approach which is vitalistic, nondeterministic and non-reductionistic, an approach which focuses on the "givens" of existence, on contingency, on meaning and purpose in life, on will, on decision and choice, on commitment, on shift in attitude and life perspective. There is no standard set of existential techniques; on the contrary, the approach is by definition nontechnique oriented. For the purpose of this discussion I consider any method I used to turn Ginny's head in the direction of these issues as an "existential technique."

What is the relationship between this approach and the development of "will"? Admittedly, unclear and unsystematic. I tried through my interpretative efforts with Ginny to remove obstacles to will, to weaken the cohorts of counter-will. I cannot describe these efforts in a trim, methodical fashion. It will have to do to say that I fertilized the soil, that I was an *accoucheur* to the birthing of will.

I tried a variety of methods to coax, urge, coerce Ginny to recognize the intrauterine kicks of her unborn will. Repeatedly I reminded her that she had both voice and choice in her future; she was responsible for herself. She gave others the right to define her but even this act was choiceful; she was not so helpless as she believed. I challenged her life perspective in a number of ways. Could she not view her current dilemmas from another vista point, from the perspective of the long skein of her life? What was core Ginny and what was peripheral—something quite extrinsic, something that would pass away, something that at the end of her life would be a meaningless speck? What of the future? In ten years did she still want to be in a loveless, barren relationship—all because she dare not speak, dare not act? And what of death? Could the knowledge of death not help her free herself from the ebbtides of basically unimportant events? I chided her or tried to shock her. "What would you like written on your tombstone? 'Here lies Ginny, flunked in her foreign language school by Mr. Flood?' Is that sufficient meaning for your life? If not then rise above it, do something about it." . . . "The everyday events consume your energy, submerge your will only when you lose perspective of your total life, only when you actually believe these events are central to your being." . . . "You can vanquish them with your own resources: you will know, if you only listen and look deep enough into yourself, that the events and your reactions to them are your vassals—you have constituted the world, the event, the reaction, they are entirely dependent upon you for their existence." . . . "Nothing occurs, nothing exists until you create it. How then can an event or a person control you?" . . . "You have willed them into being, you have given them power over you, and you can take away that power because it belongs to you. Everything emanates from your will."

Sometimes I thought of myself as raining upon Ginny's tin roof. I wanted to pour, to fling sheets of water from all directions at once. I wanted to drench her. But I had to restrain myself lest I succeed only in establishing a neural anastomosis in which Ginny's body would obey my every wish. A psychotherapeutic Catch-22: Do what I suggest, but do it for yourself!

In addition to "interpretative" and "existential" techniques, there was a third major facet to my therapy with Ginny. I call it "activation" but it could go by other names: behaviorial modification, behavioral manipulation, desensitization, deconditioning, etc. To describe this part of my work does not please me, I take little pride in

227

it, it is demeaning to me and to Ginny. She loses her dignity, she becomes thingish, an object whose behavior I must modify. And yet there are those who will claim that any change that occurred in Ginny was mediated primarily and precisely through these techniques. And the arguments they can muster will be compelling ones.

So we must get on with it. Behaviorial therapy is an approach to change based on learning theory. More mechanistic even than instinct-based psychoanalysis, it ignores insight, self-knowledge, consciousness, meaning—in short much that constitutes the very essence of our humanness. Not that there is an explicit conspiracy to dehumanize man; it is only that these factors, so a behaviorist would claim, are largely irrelevant to the process of change. Learning takes place in man, as in lower orders of life, according to certain explicit and quantifiable processes—by operant conditioning (the reward, extinction, or punishment of certain behaviors); by modeling (imitation of some valued individual); by principles of classical conditioning (the temporal or spatial approximation of a critical stimulus and an indifferent one); by an active trial and error stance in contrast to a passive or receptive attitude. Psychopathology is learned behavior which is maladaptive and rigid. Psychotherapy, a process of unlearning old behaviors and learning new ones, proceeds according to the rigorous tenets of learning theory.

To explicate let us consider briefly the application of these techniques. Imagine that a patient has a single, well circumscribed problem: an irrational fear of snakes. Imagine, too, that since he is a gardener, the symptom is a disabling one and his motivation for therapy is high. A behaviorial therapist would gradually expose the patient to the feared stimulus in situations in which he could experience little anxiety. Profound muscular relaxation blocks the development of strong anxiety. Therefore, while in a state of deep muscular relaxation, often induced hypnotically, the patient is asked to imagine looking at a picture of a snake, then perhaps to imagine seeing a snake one hundred feet away, then closer, then to look at a picture of a snake and finally after several hours to see a snake, and then perhaps to handle one. The principle is simple: exposure to stimuli previously regarded as dangerous under situations so safe that the fear response is inhibited. If repeated many times the stimulus-fear sequence is extinguished and the new learning is transferred out of the laboratory or therapist's office back to the home situation. Modeling is also encouraged; for example the therapist may take walks with the patient on high grassy lawns, or may handle a snake in the patient's presence.

I have over-simplified the procedure by using an elementary paradigm, but for our purposes it is sufficient. Consider now how learning theory techniques pervaded my work with Ginny. She had an irrational fear (a phobia, if you will) of self-assertion. She acted as if some calamity would ensue were she to demand her rights or express anger or merely a conflicting opinion.

Our testing laboratory was to be our relationship; I attempted to establish an environment of such trust, nonjudgmental acceptance and mutual respect that the fear response would be inhibited. Then I proceeded to expose Ginny to the dreaded stimulus as I encouraged her in graduated steps to assert herself with me. The encouragement took many forms from coaxing, counsel, and persuasion to model setting, demands and ultimatums. At times I was a playful, cajoling uncle, or a persistent Socratic gadfly, or a stern, demanding director, or a second in a boxing match resolutely inspiriting Ginny from behind a post in a corner of the ring. I wanted her to emerge, to ask me questions, to demand that I be on time, to request a more convenient hour, to contradict me, to be angry with me, to express her disappointment with me. I put words in her mouth: "If I were you, I would feel. . . ." When the assertiveness emerged, and it came slowly and feebly, I welcomed it ("reinforced" it, if you must). Transfer of learning or generalization was the next task. I proceeded to urge her to take some small steps with Karl. I role played Karl with her, we rehearsed imaginary mini-confrontations ranging from such issues as gas money, to housekeeping chores to sexual foreplay.

Each of these assertive forays was reinforced not only by my acceptance but by the nonappearance of the fantasied holocaust. Each hitherto dangerous act was made safer by the safety of my office. Then the great step outward: our meetings together with Karl. Potentially dangerous, of course, but still less risky than the same confrontation without my presence.

There was, of course, far more behaviorial modification than desensitization to the fear of self-assertion. Ginny could not be "herself" in so many other ways. She could be accepted or loved only by acting or performing, she could not voice her despair, her fear of disintegration, her deep sense of emptiness, her love. I asked her to

229

show me everything. Try me, I said, I will stay with you, listen to you, accept you in your entirety.

Therapy viewed in this way was a carefully scripted dress rehearsal, an exercise in deterrorfication, an enterprise whose task it was to make itself unnecessary, to extinguish itself. But of course it was more. It refused to accept its fate. The frame dissolved, the actors began to exist in their roles, the director refused to remain a behavioral engineer.

* * *

So much for the theory behind my therapy with Ginny, for the techniques and their rationale. I have delayed as long as I can. What about the therapist, me, the other actor in this drama? In my office I hide behind my title, interpretations, my Freudian beard, penetrating gaze and posture of ultimate helpfulness; in this book, behind my explanations, my thesaurus, my reportorial and belletristic efforts. But this time I have gone too far. If I do not step gracefully out of my sanctum sanctorum, almost certainly my analytic-colleague reviewers will yank me out.

The issue, of course, is countertransference. During our life together Ginny often related to me irrationally, on the basis of a very unrealistic appraisal of me. But what of my relationship to her? To what extent did my own unconscious or barely conscious needs dictate my perception of Ginny and my behavior toward her?

It is not entirely true that she was the patient and I the therapist. I first discovered that a few years ago when I spent a sabbatical year in London. I had no claims on my time and had planned to do nothing but work on a book on group therapy. Apparently that was not enough; I grew depressed, restless and finally arranged to treat two patients—more for my sake than for theirs. Who was the patient and who the therapist? I was more troubled than they, and, I think benefited more than they from our work together.

For over fifteen years, I have been a healer; therapy has become a core part of my self-image; it provides me meaning, industry, pride, mastery. Thus, Ginny helped me by allowing me to help her. But I had to help her a great deal, a very great deal. I was Pygmalion, she my Galatea. I had to transform her, to succeed where others had failed, and to succeed in an astonishingly brief period of time.

(Though this book may seem lengthy, sixty hours is a relatively short course of therapy.) The miracle worker. Yes, I own that, and the need was not silent in therapy: I pressured her relentlessly, I gave voice to my frustration when she rested or consolidated for even a few hours, I improvised continuously. "Get well," I shouted at her, "get well for your sake, not for your mother's sake or for Karl's—get well for yourself." But, very softly, I also said, "get well for me, help me be a healer, a rescuer, a miracle worker." Did she hear me? I scarcely heard myself.

In still another more evident way the therapy was for me. I became Ginny and treated myself. She was the writer I always wanted to become. The pleasure I obtained from reading her sentences transcended sheer aesthetic appreciation. I struggled to unlock her, to unlock myself. How many times during therapy did I go back twenty-five years to my high school English class, to old frayed Miss Davis who read my compositions aloud to the class, to my embarrassing notebooks of verse, to my never-begotten Thomas Wolfe-ian novel. She took me back to a crossroad, to a path I never dared take for myself. I tried to take it through her. "If only Ginny could have been deeper," I said to myself. "Why did she have to be content with satire and parody? What I could have done with that talent!" Did she hear me?

The healer-patient, the rescuer, Pygmalion, the miracle worker, the great unrealized writer. Yes, all these. And there is more. Ginny developed a strong positive transference toward me. She overvalued my wisdom, my potency. She fell in love with me. I tried to work with that transference, to "work through" it, to resolve it in a therapeutically beneficial way. But I had to work against myself as well. I *want* to appear wise and omnipotent. It is important that attractive women fall in love with me. And so in my office we were many patients sitting in many chairs. I struggled against parts of myself, trying to ally with parts of Ginny in the conflict against other parts. I had to monitor myself continuously. How many times did I silently ask myself, "Was that for me or for Ginny?" Often I caught myself engaging or about to engage in a seduction that would do nothing but foster Ginny's exaltation of me. How many times did I elude my own watchful eye?

I became far more important to Ginny than she to me. It is so with every patient, how could it be otherwise? A patient has only one therapist, a therapist many patients. And so Ginny dreamt about me, held imaginary conversations with me during the week (just as I used to converse with my analyst, old Olive Smith—bless her staunch heart), or imagined I was there at her elbow watching her every action. And yet there is more to it. True, Ginny rarely entered my fantasy life. I did not think about her between sessions, I never dreamed about her, yet I know that I cared deeply about her. I think I did not permit myself full knowledge of my feelings and so I must awkwardly deduce these things about myself. There were many clues: my jealousy toward Karl; my disappointment when Ginny missed a session; my snug, cozy feelings when we were together ("snug" and "cozy" are just the right words—not clearly sexual but by no means ethereal). All these are self-evident, I expected and recognized them, but what was unexpected was the eruption of my feelings when my wife moved into my relationship with Ginny. Earlier I described our social meeting in California after the end of therapy. When Ginny left I was morose, diffusely irritated and sullenly refused my wife's invitations to talk about our meeting. Though my phone conversations with Ginny were generally brief and impeccably professional, I was invariably uneasy at my wife's presence in the room. It is even possible that I invited, ambivalently, my wife into our relationship to help me with my counter-transference. (I am not sure, though; my wife generally helps me in editing my work.) All these reactions become explicable if one concludes that I was in the midst of a heavily sublimated affair with Ginny.

Ginny's positive transference complicated therapy in many ways. I wrote earlier that she was in therapy in large part to be with me. To get well was to say goodbye. "And so she remained suspended in a great selfless wasteland, not so well as to lose me, not so sick as to drive me away in frustration." And I? What did I do to prevent Ginny from leaving me? This book has insured that Ginny never will become a half-forgotten name in my old appointment book or a lost voice on an electromagnetic band. In both a real and symbolic sense we have defeated termination. Would it be going too far to say that our affair has been consummated in this shared work?

Add then Lothario, lover, to the list of healer-patient, rescuer, Pygmalion, unborn writer, and still there is more which I cannot or will not see. Countertransference was always present, like a gauzed veil through which I attempted to see Ginny. To the best of my ability I tugged at it, I stared through it, I refused, as best I could, to allow it to obstruct our work. I know that I did not always succeed, nor am I convinced that the total subjugation of my irrational side, needs and wishes would have promoted therapy; in a bewildering fashion countertransference supplied much of the energy and humanity that made our venture a successful one.

Was therapy successful? Has Ginny undergone substantial change? Or do we see "a transference cure," she having merely learned how to behave differently, how to appease and please the now-internalized Dr. Yalom? The reader shall have to judge for himself. I feel satisfied with our work and optimistic about Ginny's progress. There are remaining areas of conflict, yet I regard them with equanimity; I have long ago lost the sense that I as the therapist have to do it all. What is important is that Ginny is unfrozen and can take an open posture to new experiences. I have confidence in her ability to continue changing and my view is supported by most objective measures.

She has now terminated a relationship with Karl which, with retrospective wisdom, was growth retarding for both parties; she is actively writing and, for the first time, functioning well in a responsible and challenging job (a far cry from the playground worker or the placard-carrying traffic guard); she has established a social circle and a more satisfying relationship with a new man. Gone are the night panics, the frightening dreams of disintegration, the migraines, the petrifying self-consciousness and self-effacement.

But I would have been satisfied even without these observable measures of outcome. I wince as I confess that, since I have devoted much of my professional career to a rigorous, quantifiable study of the outcome of psychotherapy. It is a paradox hard to embrace, even harder to banish. The "art" of psychotherapy has for me a dual meaning: "art" in that the execution of therapy requires the use of intuitive faculties not derivable from scientific principles and "art" in the Keatsian sense that it establishes its own truth transcending objective analysis. The truth is a beauty that Ginny and I experienced. We knew one another, touched one another deeply, and shared splendid moments not easily come by.

March 1, 1974

233

Ginny's Afterword

KARL AND I had been together for eight months in the new state and had rarely connected in a personal way. My world got smaller and smaller. Karl would go off on trips; he found colleagues. He led his life away from the house. Occasionally our similar sensibilities, sense of humor and dinner would put us side by side. But even when we spent a lot of time together, it was as inanimate objects—like a chair and couch next to each other in a hotel lobby. Karl would have to be questioned before he would tell me anything about his day or give me anything. He even withheld his wonderful fault—the long stories of his day. And my conversation seemed to come out of nowhere since in the day I had been nowhere. I was fearful, sure that Karl sensed the claustrophobia of my mind and tension.

I accepted my boundaries growing smaller and smaller. But I began to feel so redundant—like I was living a part of my life again and again—never getting beyond it. I was loving my man only slightly, losing him in our oblivion. I still didn't have a job, just freelance bouts with writing; my discipline was only seasonal (when it was warm and lovely, I headed for a kid's type of existence). The days got old real fast and then hung on long and ominous. I was living a miniature life as a hardened dreamer, and feeling ashamed, apologetic, because the circumference of my life was about the size of a marble. Hours of day and night accumulated against me.

I had an aversion to life. Before, in the mornings I used to wake up fast and lively like a latent farmhand, but lately I had dreamt of milking my own blood out, of not having to go on. That brink which I had seemed constantly mounted on, became a wall. I rebelled by fantasies of writing, leaving, living strongly alone—the usual. Building continuous dialogues out of silence. Using my love life with Karl and dragging it into fuller dreams at night while he was asleep. All the while my real voice in the real world diminished.

235

Karl and I seemed to have quit dalliance so fast. There were no anticipations. You get bored or ready to leave listening to a clock tick. Well Karl and I were like clockwork.

It wasn't always that way. Dr. Yalom had really given us a generosity and hope toward each other. Back in California when Karl was trying to survive in life without the curriculum of a job or any pay check prestige, I remember he used to often go to the library and try to write. Once he brought back a page of his aims and (small victory) he read them to me. There were no aims and only a few thin innuendos that had anything to do with positioning me in his life. (This after over two years together.) It hurt me and I spoke to him about it. I didn't betray what I wanted to say even though I watered it down with a few tears. I wanted to be part of his life and not just a few years of shared rent. I wanted something with him that changed from day to day, something that he thought about and cared for. Not just a duffel bag that he remembered when he was moving.

Because we had had that moment of sharing—he, his writing; me, my anguish—he promised me that the good days were ahead and then, you know, I thought they were. Anyway there was a good night ahead when we played liar dice on green felt, and I won. And we ate a second dinner about 11:30 and smoked and ate yogurt and listened to music. And touched each other a long time and made love. And I responded and felt wonderful. But just stayed this side of consciousness a long time and felt sad, which is a euphemism. I never could break out of the pattern by completely relaxing or forgetting. And I thought bitterly —"ridiculous me, always on some brink." My mind was definitely top heavy and would not give its consent to my body. I couldn't get off of the tread mill that haunted my mind during sex and life with Karl.

The days just got worse, more oblivious. I had reserved no real time for any destination or goal that required my own abilities alone. I'd chosen to be a lizard in the desert, flattered by the sun. Only I had human nerves and wits. I had been living tongue-in-cheek and withering. And my panics at night increased and didn't drizzle off in the morning. My mind let out a stampede on my body. I lay helpless, sacrificed until daylight rounded the feelings up, then my bruised body could leave. These panics

I'm sure were caused by the lack of hope between Karl and me, and the knowledge that soon I would be abandoned. (If I tried to conjure up Dr. Yalom at these times, it was only to put him into my melodrama.)

Even Karl's judgmental side waned into apathy. He ignored me. I could talk back to him on factual matters, stand up in that way thanks to Dr. Yalom, but I couldn't demand feelings. I couldn't ask him about our future. As John Prine says, "A question ain't really a question, if you know the answer too." * I was fearful; Karl sensed my tension. But I think it was the truth that was tensing me. You have to do all the emotions when you're the only one involved in a relationship. There was no intuition on Karl's part. I was trumping up love songs and come-ons. Whole nights of snuggling and near misses. I could be close at night when he was unconscious.

I guess I lost track of who Karl was. Not that he left many tracks around the house worth following. They all led to work. There was just no give. Karl was as good as anyone in terms of fun, of talks, games and latent sensitivity, but he narrowed his compass terribly: in fact, just downright sliced off a few directions. And I followed, not allowing my wants to impinge, to influence him, to lighten our life.

I was like a needy child with a cruel stepfather; the situation was ridiculous. I was standing up to offer him my seat but he was getting off at the next stop anyhow.

Finally, desperate, unable to consume my own silence and the shared resistance to our life together, I said, "Karl, we're not getting along worth a shit." And he said, "I know. I want out. I'm burnt out." And by the next night he was gone.

* * *

Karl is gone. But this is not the day that my life came apart, it is just the echo finally returning from a long severing cry. I'm scared. I can't eat and I wouldn't take odds on the sleep

---

* "Far from Me," © copyright 1971 by Cotillion Music & Sour Grapes Music. Used by permission.

that lies before me. I've tried to separate what was just need, dependence and appliances from what were real feelings and love for Karl. The radio, T.V., books, his; plus the silence, greed, laughter, car rides. I'm trying to get an honest feeling about Karl that is not jumbled up with necessities and nausea. And trying to feel that my own presence exists.

Karl's presence is still about me—his name still sounds familiar, not far away, not years gone. I still quote him and know his desires and qualms. I am sure that Karl was not just a habit. The piano was a habit. I gave it up after seven years—no tears. Sometimes Karl's leaving is a feeling and sometimes a reality. Most times it's a sadness that exists without being born of any particular fact. After several weeks, though, I realized I couldn't stay at this level of just perfect perception of a painful situation. Karl will not come back; it will not happen, even if unwisely I wish it with my whole being (we know how whole that is). I wake up from dreams where Karl has been active in taunting me; losing him in my sleep as I lost him in my life.

This time of sadness and utter dampness became uninhabitable. I knew I only had a death wish and a death sentence to choose, if I let timidity and condemnation hold me to this spot of rejection. The space where my smile used to be felt fractured. Anyway too much of my grief was self-inflicted and well deserved—the backlash of years of standing still and waiting. Leading a clean life as an empty slate. Karl's leaving was too connected to the emptiness and boredom of my life to be wholly pure and sentimentalized.

I'm scared because always I've thought of myself as buried except for the fingertips of friends and chance talky acquaintances helping and laughing with me. So I've always had to station myself where I could be bumped into, and part of Karl was meeting people with him. I could live by carefully tossed-out asides and clever ideas. I felt if I ever lost my positioning, just a few degrees askew of the mainstream, that no one would ever see me again, that I would lose all chance.

And in fact I have given my life up to chance till now. I have shivered in fear and grown in my trances. And now if life is to go with me at all, I must get out and live, not wait. It seems all I did was give my energy to the minutes, while waiting for the next coincidence. (Coincidence—a good name for a horse that will win once in-a-while but mostly lose.) I put all my soul on pass, watching someone else be the mover and thrower.

Now I have to move, go ahead with an out-going unginny life, as Dr. Yalom might say. A life where I don't use mediators to cushion and introduce me to and from the world; don't knock into dreams when I'm doing the simplest things, and try to engage in forthright conversations in which my loose ends aren't coyly used to flagellate and downgrade me. No one can delve into my brain and bring out some thinking, no one but me.

I realized the difference between thinking and what I'd been doing spontaneously for so long—worrying. In worrying, I only mulled over the bad alternatives. Thinking is progressive, extending. I never did it. And fantasying is still-life thinking, knowing you're never going to do anything about your visions. I'd been used to letting people handle the pragmatic side of life, while I became a genius at tangents.

No man will ever choose to live with my osmosis till death do us part. I will have to inhabit myself or there will be nothing there. No, now I must move aggressively and without any magic tunes or coincidences. I am just ordinary.

* * *

Life became hard; there was no love life to soften it. However, even by the standards of the most over stretched soap opera, the mourning time was over. But I sometimes said stupid things that were consoling instead of getting on with it. "I shall not see Karl again with his eyes closed or touch his sleep in the morning." But if I were to stay crying and nuzzling souvenirs of Karl's and my time together, I'd be like a steady teenager going around and round a dead top ten.

I've skipped the final beat of recognition that Karl is never coming back; I've also lost an inch of soft clouds that padded my brain and kept it from perfect sighting of distress, but also happiness. Glacier-like tears that will take months to make their way down my mind are still there, but I forget them. I don't cry much anymore. I try to ignore a growing nostalgia for those tears. There is more silence and the few tears are surrounded by anger.

Pain, I got to know you, and I'm not going to waste any more precious time with you. How frustrating for Dr. Yalom to hear me ranting and raving over the glories of tears and nightmares. I'm not going to try to define myself any more by pain and tears. I don't need them to make me human. I never want to follow this circle again.

Besides, deep down, past the desperate feelings of abandonment, there is a feeling of rightness, that I really wished for Karl and me not to be together, that I had wanted to get out, seethed with it, hoped for his decision, but as usual, a staggering inertia made up of pity and fear had kept me in the situation.

*   *   *

> Every day seems a little longer
> Every way love's a little stronger
> Come what may, do you ever long for true love
> from me?
>
> Love like yours will surely come my way.*

Strangely now I am more reconciled to the loss of Karl than to the finality of my time with Dr. Yalom, even though I never really gave in to therapy. I never completely believed in the emaciated self I brought into Dr. Yalom's life each week. Because I knew that on the outside (the real world) I could be sort of vivacious and dramatic and happy and had several wonderful, long-time long believing friends. And I'd had normal and almost normal talks and days with Karl. But I did not want to give up the part of me which touched Dr. Yalom because it seemed what little I said there was more resonant and had deeper echoes than any quips and puns I spun off ouside. Often I played dead, but whether I was dead silly or just dead, I still had a lightness, optimism and lease on life and knew it. I never allowed much pain.

At times I acted in his office, deliberately subduing my spirit

---

* "Every Day," by Norman Petti and Charles Hardin, © copyright 1957 by Peer International Corporation. Used by permission.

to coincide with the therapy hour. I could be mock indignant, but never angry. Yet I did want to dig down and strike something real, something in me that could initiate and not just tag along. Some emotional geyser, instead of our vaudeville patter, with Dr. Yalom using his psychiatrist's hook, and me my self-conscious back-talk, to pull the curtain down.

The write-ups too were sometimes deliberately somber and serious or sloppy and fluffy. I seemed to have no other jargon but what was already in me; I couldn't force myself to reach for the healing words he wanted; I couldn't have Clinical Mouth and answer his questions in kind; give the straight psychiatrist's party line. Every time Dr. Yalom asked me a healing question, I'd be quiet, or worse, grin. Because I knew how easy it would be to resort to my old self; I wanted to find something new, something other than the stamina of nerves and illusions that clothed me.

I didn't defend myself. In a sense I let the scenario be written by others and then followed, hearing many cues but delivering only a few lines. One of Dr. Yalom's most predictable questions was, "What do you like about me, or Karl, or yourself?" That question was almost as far away as the other side of the coin, "Ginny, isn't there anything you object to in me?"

I knew he was trying to draw me to reality, and I suppose I even knew reality, but it had no impact on me. I can't bear to look at people objectively, though I don't mind swatting at them with metaphors. It is easier for me to adapt and accept than judge. I hate to distance people by limiting them to their roles, like "mother," "father," "psychiatrist"—each person has his own particular justifications. I guess I could defend them all, even at my own expense, in my stillness, because it hurts more to put them down, to hate them.

*　*　*

I think I achieved something personal with you, Dr. Yalom. You tried to bind it up in a ribbon of therapy, and I was always a little suspicious, or worse, sarcastic (takes less energy) about what you fed me, even though I said I was starving.

I feel there will always be a whole unreconciled area, a gap in therapy—that our aims were different. You could not know how it felt to be blank or, on the other side of the coin, vivaciously alive and inspired. The times I was free made me realize that my goal should always be to seek that feeling of warmth, of no subconscious corners, of straightness. The answers to your direct questions sometimes didn't seem to be my answers. I wasn't interested in a hierarchy of questions and answers. All the time I was not really searching for change but for a man whom I could talk to as I did to you, who would question and understand me, have your patience, and yet be separate from me.

Dr. Yalom, you always rooted for me, trying to get me out of low tide and back into the flow of things. I watched you, fascinated at times, but when I got out of your vision, there was so little current. Now I draw you around me again, like small waves, and the illusion is that I am moving, and not grafted to the stillness of dusk or the impression of sand.

Actually I think that simile and metaphor and all the ones I threw at you in my reports and talk (all five billion) are one thing and I'm another. I used them as a veil, until I could talk directly to you.

* * *

I didn't stay down for the full count of suffering. Maybe I don't have the guts to be knocked out totally. I can only fantasize that moment. (After all the premonitions and previews I gave you of what would happen to me if I were ever truly abandoned, maybe the least I could have done is expire.)

For a month I did live a private, painful life. But by the end of that time, the resilient streak in me was up. I found out that the friends I had were still around me. All that was missing was Karl's deadening presence and unhappiness.

I am now mid-way through a day with no close feelings of anxiety. I've gotten a job doing some research and writing, thanks to others who helped me. It's no salvation but gives me money, so I can stop stockpiling a few promises of things I should do but can't afford. I've always drizzled my money away, not using it to see any future or goals. Healthy people seem to reach out and hold more and more of life while withdrawn people such as myself, hold less and less of life.

I've got to change that—I can feel the distance I must go. Friends become scary as I realize I cannot be just a presence, a spirit, all my life. My friends are saying that they want more of me. These are some of the messages that Karl gave me, only there seems more love and giving in the bargain. Of course, all these changes make me grit my teeth since challenge freezes me still. I know I need more than a few declarative sentences and some marching music. Practically every task must be brought up to a human level. My best friends tell me to choose my words and deal with things more chronologically and make choices. Try for an unginny life.

Not only have I stopped suffering, but despite my initial resistance, I've met another man. I'm surprised how quickly the past has stopped. He cares for me and is attracted to me. And I am attracted to him, in fact, cannot keep my hands off him. I really find myself feeling more like a woman and less like a girl. My brain is much less calculating and is more at home with voices than the mere echoes and dreams I used to feed it. I have confidence that registers as warm flashes in my stomach and a constant energy. The fear and dread are gone. Maybe they have turned into irony which at least is softer and not so flattening. In any case, irony is flimsy stuff compared to the good days I am having.

There are still plenty of problems though. I feel my life is contingent on certain securities—having my own nest, some money, my new friend whom I want to see often, and a close girlfriend who is precious to my life, as close as a shadow. And I still am disorganized; the kitchen table spreads out over a whole floor, a whole room. I feel scattered a lot of times, both in terms of possessions springing out of closets and in things to do.

Maybe things will grow bad. Then I can fight back. I only got smaller by shrinking away from problems and burdening you with my silence. I want to achieve something personal in my life, not always go after the performance. My mind feels really slack as though it had studied the world through a series of mirages, which I tried to describe dutifully to you, Dr. Yalom.

Now when I rake my brain for some factual matter, I wish I had tried to talk more, even if it weren't all pure, instead of holding out for the sentence whose emotion was one hundred proof.

I stared off into a lot of space in your office, going back and forth in time and not settling. Now I feel sure I could find your face and so find mine, and talk clearly or be quiet. You are the you understood of these pages.

The brokenness of yesterday is patched. My pain is perennial but so is my happiness.

In your office I was stringing jokes like worry beads through my fingers. I was happy just for your company (which was always natural and giving) but I was scared to live like other people. I didn't really want a therapist's office, but a nest; I tried to pull you down into my hibernation and helpless calm. You didn't let me succeed at just nodding or pretending to dream. When your art succeeded, you revived us both.

As often as I curled up, you uncurled me.

March 1, 1974